ALCOHOL

ALCOHOL

Peter L. Myers and Richard E. Isralowitz

Health and Medical Issues Today

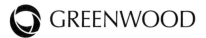 GREENWOOD

AN IMPRINT OF ABC-CLIO, LLC
Santa Barbara, California • Denver, Colorado • Oxford, England

Library of Congress Cataloging-in-Publication Data

Myers, Peter L.
    Alcohol / Peter L. Myers and Richard E. Isralowitz.
        p. ; cm. — (Health and medical issues today)
    Includes bibliographical references and index.
    ISBN 978-0-313-37247-6 (hardback : alk. paper) — ISBN 978-0-313-37248-3
(ebook)   1. Alcohol—Toxicology.   2. Alcohol—Physiological effect.
3. Alcoholism—Complications.   4. Drinking of alcoholic beverages—Social aspects.
I. Isralowitz, Richard.   II. Title.   III. Series: Health and medical issues today.
    [DNLM: 1. Alcohol-Related Disorders.   2. Alcohol Drinking.   3. Cost of Illness.
4. Public Policy.   5. Socioeconomic Factors.   WM 274]
    RA1242.A35M94   2011
    615'.7828—dc22   2011002182

ISBN: 978-0-313-37247-6
EISBN: 978-0-313-37248-3

15 14 13 12 11   1 2 3 4 5

This book is also available on the World Wide Web as an eBook.
Visit www.abc-clio.com for details.

Greenwood
An Imprint of ABC-CLIO, LLC

ABC-CLIO, LLC
130 Cremona Drive, P.O. Box 1911
Santa Barbara, California 93116-1911

This book is printed on acid-free paper ∞

Manufactured in the United States of America

To my mother, Helen, my children, and, in
memory, my father, Sam.
—*REI*

To the newest member of the family, the wonderful
Zane Samuel Rizvi.
—*PLM*

CONTENTS

SERIES FOREWORD

Every day, the public is bombarded with information on developments in medicine and health care. Whether it is on the latest techniques in treatments or research, or on concerns over public health threats, this information directly affects the lives of people more than almost any other issue. Although there are many sources for understanding these topics—from Web sites and blogs to newspapers and magazines—students and ordinary citizens often need one resource that makes sense of the complex health and medical issues affecting their daily lives.

The *Health and Medical Issues Today* series provides just such a one-stop resource for obtaining a solid overview of the most controversial areas of health care in the twenty-first century. Each volume addresses one topic and provides a balanced summary of what is known. These volumes provide an excellent first step for students and lay people interested in understanding how health care works in our society today.

Each volume is broken into several sections to provide readers and researchers with easy access to the information they need:

- Part I provides overview chapters on background information—including chapters on such areas as the historical, scientific, medical, social, and legal issues involved—that a citizen needs to intelligently understand the topic.
- Part II provides capsule examinations of the most heated contemporary issues and debates, and analyzes in a balanced manner the viewpoints held by various advocates in the debates.

- Part III provides a selection of reference material, such as annotated primary source documents, a timeline of important events, and a directory of organizations that serve as the best next step in learning about the topic at hand.

The *Health and Medical Issues Today* series strives to provide readers with all the information needed to begin making sense of some of the most important debates going on in the world today. The series includes volumes on such topics as stem-cell research, obesity, gene therapy, alternative medicine, organ transplantation, mental health, and more.

PREFACE AND ACKNOWLEDGMENTS

On July 30, 2009, four men sat at a table on the White House lawn to drink beer: President Barack Obama, Vice President Joe Biden, noted African American historian Professor Henry Louis Gates of Harvard University, and Sgt. James Crowley of the Cambridge, Massachusetts, police force. Crowley had arrested and handcuffed Gates in his own home just 10 days earlier, touching off a national furor on racial profiling. The so-called beer summit was photographed, discussed, and dissected on blogs and newscasts and in barbershops and bars nationwide. With a drink, the president hoped to symbolically bridge a racial divide.

The toxicology examiner of Westchester County, New York, stated that Diane Schuler was swigging vodka and had a blood-alcohol concentration of more than twice the legal limit on July 26, 2009, when she drove past two Do Not Enter signs onto the Taconic State Parkway and continued two miles into oncoming traffic before smashing head-on into an SUV, killing herself; her 2-year-old daughter; nieces ages 5, 7, and 9; and the three occupants of the SUV. In response to what seemed an epidemic of mothers driving drunk that summer, the New York State legislature passed a law on November 17 making it a felony to drive drunk with children in the car. Many commentators reiterated the public-health message that drunk drivers have difficulty with their perception, judgment, memory, and peripheral vision, as well in the motor skills involved in driving. Clearly, not everyone was listening: At a tavern also near the Taconic State Parkway in August 2010, a woman wove over to the jukebox, selecting Toby Keith's "I Love This Bar" and "Whiskey Girl" and George Thorogood's "I Drink Alone" and his version (Thorogood, 2007) of the 1953 blues ballad "One Bourbon, One Scotch, One Beer" (Toombs, 1953). She later drove off, clearly inebriated. While the fate of this individual is unknown to us, we do know that in Suffolk County, New York, there were six arrests for wrong-way, drunken highway driving between November 15 and December 15, 2010, alone.

The paradox of alcohol: It is a celebratory and ceremonial social beverage, woven throughout the fabric of society and culture. Even the common man is called Joe Six-Pack. Yet globally, alcohol accounts for 1 out of 25 deaths annually (Rehm et al., 2009). To provide but one example, during the severe heat wave of 2010 in Russia, thousands of Russians drowned while swimming intoxicated. Alcohol misuse incurs billions of dollars in costs to society annually through medical, insurance, and criminal-justice costs and time lost in the workplace.

To understand even the Schuler tragedy, we need to understand the blood chemistry of alcohol, the effects of alcohol on the nervous system, a consideration of what would motivate a mother to drive drunk, and the contexts of family and community and of politics and culture within which alcohol is consumed. Doing so necessitates that we draw on multiple professional disciplines in compiling this brief reference volume.

Alcohol, of course, is only one of the many psychoactive chemicals that people use, although it is the most widely used. To round out the picture of chemical abuse and addiction, readers may want to consult our companion volume in this series, *Illicit Drugs*.

ACKNOWLEDGMENTS

Richard E. Isralowitz wishes to express profound gratitude to Sofia Borkin, MD, for her unwavering support of our efforts.

Peter L. Myers wishes to express profound gratitude to Susan Briggs Myers, LCSW, for her continuing support of our efforts.

The authors wish to thank David Paige, Mike Nobel, and Michelle Scott of ABC-CLIO and the team at Apex CoVantage for their help, expertise, and patience.

PART I

History and Scientific Background

Alcohol: An Overview

CHAPTER 1

Alcohol: The Basics

WHAT IS ALCOHOL?

Alcohols are a class of volatile, flammable organic compounds with a wide variety of uses. (See "The Other Alcohols," below.) In everyday language, *alcohol* refers to beverage alcohol that is ethyl alcohol or ethanol. Ethanol has the chemical formula C_2H_5OH, showing that it has two carbon atoms, six hydrogen atoms, and one oxygen atom. Figure 1.1 is a simplified diagram of the chemical structure of ethanol.

Ethanol is the most widely used psychoactive drug and intoxicant. Ethanol-based beverages are drunk by a majority of people in most nations, except for those that practice Islam.

Ethanol acts as a depressant to many central nervous system functions, including judgment, reasoning, fine and gross motor skills, perception, and memory, and as a disinhibitor of behavior and emotions. At very high doses, it depresses vital bodily functions, such as respiration, with deadly effect.

Ethanol is an irritant and a toxin to tissues and organs of the body, including the esophagus, the stomach, the liver, and the pancreas. The warm feeling generated by drinking whiskey is the irritant effect of ethanol on the esophagus and the stomach.

Although beer has some nutritive value, almost all alcoholic beverages provide only empty calories. (An ounce of ethanol contains 210 calories.) The liver will preferentially oxidize ethanol over other normal nutrients, so drinking heavily tends to prevent good nutrition.

Aside from intoxicating beverages, alcohols are used in flavorings and perfumes, as solvents in medicines and various chemical compounds, as medical antiseptics and hand sanitizers, and as fuels for cooking and heating. Ethanol is also a gasoline additive that reduces hydrocarbon,

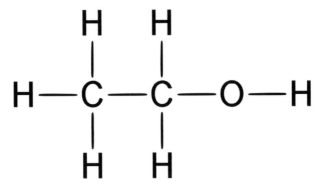

Figure 1.1   Chemical structure of ethanol (beverage alcohol).

benzene, and particulate-matter emissions that result from combustion. Controversy persists over claims that growing corn, the primary source of ethanol, to produce the additive contributes to global warming, wastes energy, and damages the environment. Ethanol is also an ingredient in some orally ingested medications. For example, Nyquil contains 25 percent ethanol.

FERMENTATION, DISTILLATION, AND TYPES OF ALCOHOLIC BEVERAGES

Alcohol is created through fermentation of carbohydrates such as sugars (found in berries and grapes) and starches (found in grains). Zymase, an enzyme in the yeast organism, catalyzes the conversion of sugars and starches into alcohol. Alcohol can also be obtained synthetically by industrial processes.

Beer and wine were the only alcoholic beverages for thousands of years until the discovery of distillation, which allowed the concentration of alcohol and thus the creation of more powerful alcoholic beverages such as rum and gin.

A typical alcoholic beverage contains half an ounce of pure ethanol. Examples include

- an 8-ounce glass of beer, at about 6 percent ethanol. (A person who says, "I don't drink much—I only drink beer" is either unaware of or equivocating about his or her alcohol intake.)
- an 8-ounce glass of wine, at 10–12 percent ethanol.

- a 1-ounce shot of hard liquor or spirits such as Scotch, Irish whiskey, brandy, gin, rye, and vodka, at 40–50 percent ethanol.
- a typical mixed drink with a 1-ounce shot of hard liquor plus a few ounces of soda or juice.

A note on mixed drinks: A complex mixed drink may contain more than one alcoholic beverage, and a few mixed drinks, such as a martini, may have two or three ounces of liquor. (Classic martini ingredients include 75 milliliters, or about 2½ ounces, of gin, 15 milliliters, or about ¼ ounces, of dry vermouth, one green olive or a twist of lemon peel, and six ice cubes.)

Alcoholic beverages may contain trace amounts of alcohols other than ethanol and other chemicals produced during manufacture. These chemicals, known as congeners, contribute to hangovers.

Types of alcoholic beverages that are the result only of fermentation include beer; wine; fortified, or dessert, wine; medicinal, or digestive, liquors; and moonshine, or home-brewed, liquors.

Beer is a product of fermenting grains, especially barley and wheat. Grains are allowed to sprout in water, releasing an enzyme that partially converts the starch into sugar. The resulting malt is boiled into a mash, allowed to ferment, and mixed with hops, a pungent herb. Beers contain 4–7 percent alcohol, except for malt liquors, which contain up to 9 percent alcohol. Most light beers contain 3.4–4.2 percent ethanol. Beers have actual nutritive value, especially from B vitamins and amino acids.

Wine is made from fermented grapes or berries crushed to extract their juices. The fermentation process occurs due to naturally occurring yeast or yeast added to the juice. Wines are allowed to age for at least six months. Wines in the United States generally have a 12–14 percent alcohol content. As of 2010, supermarkets and drugstores in many states are permitted to sell special so-called wine products with only 6–7 percent ethanol. However, In July and August 2010, supermarkets in Pennsylvania tested wine-vending kiosks, which will conduct a Breathalyzer test and a driver's license check in a pilot project that will dispense regular-strength wine. Wine coolers are another wine product, diluted with juices, that contain about 4–6 percent alcohol.

Fortified wines, including sherry, marsala, vermouth, and port, have pure alcohol or brandy added. These products are usually sweeter than regular white or red wine and have an alcoholic content of 17–21 percent. Cheap fortified wines with brands such as Night Train Express, MD 20/20 (nicknamed Mad Dog) Cisco, Wild Irish Rose, and Thunderbird are associated with subcultures of homeless alcoholics.

Fermentation cannot obtain a concentration of alcohol higher than 14 percent because ethanol will simply kill off the yeast organisms responsible for fermentation. Around A.D. 800, Arab scientists discovered a method of concentrating alcohol in liquids by evaporating some of the water, a process known as distillation, for medical purposes. Distilled spirits, or powerful alcoholic beverages, became available around A.D. 1500. These beverages, which generally contain 40–50 percent ethanol, include brandy, distilled from wine; rum, distilled from molasses or sugar cane (overproof rum may contain 75 percent ethanol); whiskeys and gin; and vodka, which is based on grain, rye, wheat, potatoes, or sugar beets.

Medicinal liquors, which often contain licorice, menthol, peppermint, or other bitters, supposedly aid digestion and suppress an upset stomach or a cough. In previous centuries, they were claimed to prevent cholera, worms, and menstrual cramps, among other ailments. Prescription of medicinal liquors (the alcohol content of which varies considerably but is generally about 40 percent) allowed manufacturers to skirt the law during the Prohibition era in the United States (1919–1933). These include brand-name drinks such as Becherovka (from the Czech Republic), Fernet Branca and Sambuca (Italy), Gammel Dansk (Denmark), Jägermeister (Germany), and Unicum (Hungary). Generic drinks in this category include the Portuguese *aguardente*, the Colombian *aguardiente*, the Chinese *gan cao*, the Greek ouzo, the French *pastis*, and the Turkish *raki*.

Bottles of distilled spirits identify the alcoholic contents according to proof, the value of which is double the percentage of ethanol in the beverage. (For example, 100 proof vodka is 50 percent ethanol.) The origins of the term, according to legend, goes back to 18th-century British naval usage. To prove that rations of rum distributed to sailors had 50 percent ethanol, a sample was added to gunpowder, which, when ignited, proved that the rum had not been watered down.

Moonshine, produced by do-it-yourself distillation, is dangerous due to contamination and other toxins present in the containers, such as old auto radiators, used to prepare the beverage (Brick, 2008, p. 1). Moonshine may also be adulterated with poisonous methanol. (See "The Other Alcohols," below.)

ALCOHOL IN THE BLOODSTREAM AND BLOOD-ALCOHOL CONCENTRATION

Ethanol, passed from the blood to tissues, is absorbed, like all nutrients, in the gastrointestinal system. Alcohol travels down the throat into the stomach, and 20 percent of ethanol is absorbed in the stomach and the rest in the duodenum and the jejunem, the first and second sections of the small intestine. Ethanol enters the capillaries of the small intestine through passive diffusion (movement from an area of higher concentration to an area of lower concentration) (Inaba & Cohen, 2007). The rate at which the stomach empties into the small intestine is an important factor in how the body absorbs ethanol, because intestinal absorption is faster. Food in the stomach slows the emptying of stomach contents, so "Don't drink on an empty stomach" is good advice. In addition, ethanol irritates and partially paralyzes the smooth stomach muscle and the pyloric valve, which leads into the small intestine, decreasing the absorption process. With high amounts of alcohol, especially on an empty stomach, the pyloric valve goes into total shutdown. The stomach, with delicate, easily irritated membranes, may send its contents back up the esophagus, which is why alcohol abusers throw up. Once alcohol has entered the bloodstream, however, it is transferred to the liver by the portal vein.

Blood-Alcohol Concentration

Blood alcohol concentration (BAC) goes up as individuals drink. Alcohol is eliminated from the body at the rate of about one drink per hour. By contrast, other drugs are eliminated gradually; half is removed from the body in a certain amount of time, and another half is removed in the same amount of time. (This is the reason for references to the half-life of a drug.)

A dose of ethanol can result, depending on the proportion of fat and water in the body, in very different BACs. Women, in general, reach a higher level of BAC than men with the same amount of ethanol, even with the same body weight, because of their higher amount of body fat as well as a smaller body mass overall.

Alcoholic beverages with a concentration of 10–30 percent ethanol are optimally absorbed. At a higher percentage, the stomach and the pyloric valve are irritated, and gastric emptying is slowed. Carbonated mixers in an alcoholic beverage result in faster absorption of alcohol (Roberts & Robinson, 2007).

BAC may be expressed in milligrams per deciliter (mg/dL) or as a percentage of alcohol in the bloodstream. A person with 100 mg/dL would have one-tenth of 1 percent of ethanol in his or her bloodstream. (This is the traditional drunk-driving limit, commonly recorded as .1, or, more accurately, $\frac{1}{10}$ of 1 percent.) Prior to the early 1990s most states defined 100 mg/dL as the drunk driving limit. Throughout the 1990s, many states lowered this to 80mg/dL, and that level became federal law in 2004. Table 1.1 summarizes the effects of various BAC levels on a person of average body mass who has not developed tolerance to the effects of alcohol.

Table 1.1 Blood Alcohol Concentration: Effects on Individuals

BAC*	Behavior	Number of Standard Drinks to Reach This Level†
.01–.05%	Decreased alertness; usually good feeling; extroversion; thought and judgment impairment; restraint loosened.	1–2
.06–.10%	Large, consistent decrease in reaction time; depth perception, distance acuity, peripheral vision, glare recovery all impaired; behavior changes; diminished awareness; small and large motor-control functions impaired.	3–4
.10%	Legally drunk; drivers can be charged with DWI.	4–5
.13–.20%	Marked depression in motor capability; decidedly intoxicated; occasional emotional demonstrations of anger, joy, weeping, shouting.	5–8
.21–.25%	Severe motor disturbances; staggering; sensory perceptions greatly impaired (e.g., blurred vision).	8–10
.30%	Semistupor. Possible alcohol poisoning.	10–15
.35%	Same consciousness level as surgical anesthesia; minimal level to cause death in some people.	10–15
.40%	Comatose.	10–15
.50%	Stopping of breathing and heartbeat possible.	10–15

*Blood-alcohol content depends on several factors, such as height, weight, and gender. Some people, including older adults, may experience alcohol effects after having fewer drinks than noted. The exact effects in older adults are not known but would be worse due to lower tolerance and increased sensitivity.

†A standard drink is a 12-ounce beer, a 4- or 5-ounce glass of wine, 1½ ounces of 80-proof liquor, or 4 ounces of liqueur. It takes about an hour to metabolize one drink. Therefore, one drink per hour is the guideline for safe drinking.

Source: Retrieved August 2010 from Substance Abuse and Mental Health Administration.

Ordinarily, intoxication accounts for about 600,000 emergency room visits in the United States each year (Pletcher, Maselli, & Gonzales, 2004). All effects of alcohol are modified in the case of a regular, heavy drinker who has developed tolerance to the presence of ethanol in the body. Notice that the root of the word *intoxication* is the same as that of *toxic*. The effects of ethanol on the brain and body, however pleasant they may feel at low doses, are actually a form of poisoning.

It is important to rule out an underlying medical condition or an emergency that can account for intoxication-like behavior such as diabetes, head injury, or stroke. Letting a supposedly drunk individual sleep it off, for example, may have fatal consequences, and emergency treatment is always a safe bet. Alternatively, alcohol intoxication may mask another dangerous medical condition. For example, an intoxicated person who gets into a car accident may have a dangerous head injury or internal bleeding. Furthermore, no specific treatment can reverse the effects of ethanol intoxication. Giving caffeine to a drunken person just results in a more alert inebriate who doesn't realize that he or she is in no position to drive.

Impairment is greater when BAC is increasing than when it falling, even for the same BAC. This is the so-called Mellanby effect, where individuals acquire tolerance during a single drinking episode (Martin & Moss, 1993). That is, if a person sits in a bar and has six drinks, raising his or her BAC to the drunk-driving limit of .08, and leaves the bar, his or her driving will be even worse than that of a person who has had ten drinks and has an BAC of .14, and sits for a while until his or her BAC is down to .08.

Blood-Alcohol Testing

The Breathalyzer and any breath-analysis test for BAC depends on ethanol diffusing from the pulmonary arterial blood into the air of the little alveolar sacs of the lung. Ethanol in one's breath compared to ethanol in the blood has a coefficient of about 2,100 to 1. Bear in mind that the test results may have to be extrapolated back from testing time to the time of an accident or the time that the subject entered the vehicle. Sucking on breath mints, eating onions, and other attempts to fool breath testing for alcohol may mask the smell but won't fool the Breathalyzer device, and the presence of mouthwash will often result in a higher BAC reading, as it commonly contains alcohol.

Among a number of breath testers, all commonly known as breathalyzers, some are designed to be preliminary breath testers that can establish probable cause for arrest of a driver, but, depending on specific state law, the results of such field tests may not be admissible in court.

Recently, several brands of personal breath testers have been marketed with the idea that the user can self-measure and know when or when not to drive. The accuracy of these personal testers varies, and some of the low-end models are not very reliable. Also, smelling alcohol on the breath is not a reliable indication of whether a person has had a drink that day. Most of the scent is from the metabolism of other chemicals in an alcoholic beverage. A person drinking pure vodka, which contains little more than water and ethanol, may have less alcohol on the breath than a beer drinker.

Metabolism and Elimination of Alcohol

Although we can often smell ethanol on the breath, or even in the sweat, of a drinker, only about 10 percent is excreted in breath, sweat, and urine. About 90 percent of ethanol is removed by oxidation, mostly in the liver. Ethanol is a nutrient with lots of calories, with an somewhere between that of carbohydrates and fats. Unlike carbohydrates and fats, however, ethanol can't be stored in the liver; it merely enters the liver and is metabolized, or broken down, there. Enzymes facilitate the breakdown of ethanol to a toxic chemical acetaldehyde, then to harmless acetic acid and eventually to carbon dioxide and water. Ethanol metabolism takes preference over the metabolism of other, normal nutrients, so one downside of drinking is the consumption of empty calories with no nutritive value. Alcohol use over time requires the drinker to consume more and more to achieve a state of intoxication; this escalation is known as tolerance. A chronic drinker can metabolize ethanol up to 72 percent faster than a nondrinker or a novice drinker.

IMMEDIATE EFFECTS OF ALCOHOL

Sleep

Millions of people use alcohol to aid in getting to sleep because it shortens the amount of time needed to enter the sleep cycle. However, the downside is that the type of sleep obtained through drinking is not the normal rhythm of the sleep cycle necessary to obtain rest; REM (rapid-eye-movement, or dream, sleep), an important part of the sleep cycle, is suppressed (Roehrs & Roth, 2001). Also, the sleeper may waken during the night, contributing to fatigue in the morning.

Kidney Function

A considerable increase in the amount of urine output occurs when BAC is elevated, especially as it is rising. This is due to the effect of alcohol on the hormone regulating the kidney. Dehydration is a direct result of increased urinary output.

The Hangover

The morning after a night in which a person has consumed several drinks is often not a happy one. *Hangover* is a general term for a collection of symptoms that may include nausea, general feelings of malaise, fatigue, and headache. There are a number of reasons for the hangover, including dehydration, because alcohol increases the rate of urine elimination, exceeding fluid intake; disturbed sleep rhythms, as described above; the toxic effect of acetaldehyde, the first breakdown product of alcohol; and ingestion of congeners, toxins in alcoholic beverages that are by-products of manufacturing, including other alcohols described in the section below. (For example, bourbon that has had its basic ethanol removed will, because of the presence of other alcohols, still provide a hangover.)

Development of Tolerance

Over time, as people drink, it will take more and more drinking to reach the desired level of intoxication, or to become impaired in cognition and motor skills. The liver gears up a more efficient burnoff of alcohol and even brings in an ancillary enzyme to help metabolize ethanol (Lieber 1999, 2004). The nervous system adapts to a certain extent as well. Finally, the chronic, heavy drinker learns behavioral stratagems to appear normal. You can mimic this by learning to talk normally with a pebble in your cheek. Some persons with alcohol use disorders, who have developed a high level of alcohol tolerance, can drive while legally drunk without apparent impairment. Individuals vary greatly in how quickly and how severely they develop some form of tolerance, and, as noted in a later section, a genetic predisposition to grow immune to the intoxicating effects of alcohol is a risk factor for development of alcohol-use disorders, as well as to the development of alcoholic liver disease. There is no great virtue in being able to drink everyone under the table.

The Other Alcohols

In general, alcohols are usually colorless, volatile (which means that they spontaneously convert to vapor), easily detected by smell, and subject to oxidation by burning—pure alcohol is highly flammable—or by metabolic oxidation within the liver.

The most important alcohols other than beverage alcohol and ethanol include methanol, or methyl alcohol (also known as wood alcohol);

isopropanol, or isopropyl alcohol (also known as rubbing alcohol); ethylene glycol; butanol or butyl alcohol; benzyl alcohol; and denatured alcohol, which is simply beverage alcohol with additives that make it undrinkable. Information about the other alcohols is important because many individuals have inadvertently ingested them for a variety of reasons, including children whose parents may not have taken care to store them safely.

Methanol, used as an industrial solvent, metabolizes to formaldehyde and formic acid and causes retinal damage, blindness, or death even if small amounts (1–2mL) are ingested (Brick 2008, p. 1). The effects may occur several hours after ingestion. Isopropanol, used as an antiseptic or as a component of an antiseptic, is so toxic that 8 ounces may be lethal. Ethylene glycol, commonly used as automotive antifreeze, has a sweet flavor but is highly poisonous, especially affecting the nervous system. The lethal dose in humans is 100 mL (3–4 ounces). Butanol is a hazardous toxic substance used for industrial purposes, including solvents and brake fluids. Benzyl alcohol, an industrial solvent, is also found in minute amounts in some medical preparations such as Anbesol, an over-the-counter anesthetic. At higher doses, however, it is toxic.

The lawyer for the Diane Schuler family, who reportedly drank 10 ounces of vodka and smoked pot behind the wheel before her wrong-way crash that killed eight people on a highway in New York State in July 2009, claimed that the driver's use of Anbesol created the postmortem alcohol-positive toxicology finding. Toxicologists, however, pointed out that while use of Anbesol immediately prior to a Breathalyzer test might provide a positive reading, the small amount of butyl alcohol it contains evaporates almost immediately, and a person would have to consume hundreds of sticks of Anbesol to exceed the legal limit for alcohol in drivers.

Finally, denatured alcohol, often written as SD alcohol (for "specially denatured), may include methanol, in which case it's known as methylated spirits, or kerosene, gasoline, other substances, or a dye. The designation SD-40 is sometimes used if the extremely bitter but not deadly substance denatonium benzoate (brand name Bitrex) is the additive. Uses of denatured alcohol include camping fuel as well as solvent or other industrial purposes. Manufacture of denatured alcohol began in the U.S. government's 1906 attempt to stop alcoholic-beverage manufacturers from avoiding the federal tax on alcohol by using industrial alcohol. By adding noxious and poisonous substances, these beverages were rendered undrinkable.

During Prohibition, however, bootleggers stole huge amounts of denatured industrial alcohol to produce illegal whiskey, often redistilling it to get rid of the adulterants. When they couldn't or didn't bother to do a perfect job, severe poisoning of drinkers ensued, especially during 1926. An article on the online magazine *Slate* by Deborah Blum (2010) claims that federal officials added toxic substances to alcohol to deliberately poison drinkers during the latter years of Prohibition, from 1926 until 1933. This claim, circulated widely on the Internet in 2010, is not found in historical accounts of that era. In fact, several years prior to that period, John Appleby, zone chief of the federal agents charged with enforcing Prohibition in New York State, warned in the *New York Times* (1922) about the diversion of denatured alcohol for beverage manufacture.

Adulteration of home-brewed spirits is a major poisoning problem in many nations, including Russia and the other nations in the former Soviet Union where home manufacture of *samagon*, or homemade vodka, is rife. High rates of alcohol-poisoning deaths in these nations, however, reflects not necessarily home-brew contamination but more often simply the lethal levels of blood alcohol achieved during drinking bouts (Stickley et al., 2007; Zaridze et al., 2009).

The consumption of all kinds of substitute alcoholic beverages during Prohibition contributed to poisoning. The 160-proof Jamaican Ginger Extract, a patent medicine nicknamed Jake, became a drink of choice in some low-income communities. It had a chemical adulterant that caused partial leg paralysis, with a resulting odd gait called jake leg or jake walk, as well as sexual impotence, informally referred to as limber trouble. The chronicling of these maladies in many blues songs was a clue that aided in tracking down the cause of this affliction.

> Aunt Jane she came runnin' and screamin', tellin' everybody
>   in the neighborhood.
> That man of mine got the limber trouble, and his lovin'
>   can't do me any good.
>   "Jake Liquor Blues," Ishmon Bracey,
>   1930

> Listen here papa, can't you see
> You can't drink jake, and get along with me
> You're a jake walkin' papa with the jake walk blues
> I'm a red hot mama that you can't afford to lose.
>   "Jake Walk Blues" Allen Brothers, 1930
>   (Baum, 2003)

Fluids and gels sold in cans for chafing dishes and camping stoves often contain poisonous alcohols. Sterno, for example, contains methanol, and Easy Heat contains diethylene glycol. According to a dangerous myth, one can strain these chafing fuels through a cloth or a loaf of bread to purify them into pure ethanol.

Alcoholics may also substitute isopropyl alcohol where alcoholic beverages are unavailable, or in quasi-suicidal behaviors. The most high-profile case in recent decades, in 1989, was that of Kitty Dukakis, wife of presidential candidate Michael Dukakis, governor of Massachusetts at the time. It was widely reported that Mrs. Dukakis was struggling with major depression and alcoholism when, under unclear circumstances, she drank rubbing alcohol (Reidy, 1990). She was briefly hospitalized, and after successful treatment for both depression and alcoholism (at the time, there was little integrated treatment for those two maladies), she became a champion of addiction-recovery causes.

CHAPTER 2

Alcohol Taken Together with Other Drugs

Beverage alcohol is a drug that can interact with many other substances we put into our bodies. Alcohol effects how other drugs work in our bodies. Even small amounts of alcohol can have an effect when taken with common, seemingly harmless drugs. While it is common to see precautions about drinking on prescription medications, alcohol taken together with acetaminophen (such as Tylenol) and aspirin can result in unwanted side effects such as liver toxicity, and liver breakdown, which is fatal. In addition, some drugs may linger in the body for days, after we assume they have cleared, so that the drug-alcohol interaction may be a stealth phenomenon.

HOW ALCOHOL AND DRUGS MAY INTERACT

The net effect of alcohol taken together with another drug may have an additive effect; three drinks and three sleeping pills, for example, equals the effect of six pills. More dangerously, it may have a multiplying or synergistic effect; three drinks and three pills equals the effect of nine pills. Drug effects may be diminished in the presence of alcohol, and a heavy drinker, even if he or she is sober, may need higher doses of medications. Alcohol may counteract a stimulant to some extent (an antagonistic effect). Furthermore, long-term use of alcohol may activate enzymes used in drug metabolism, decreasing drug availability and effects. This effect may persist for weeks even after alcohol use is stopped. When alcohol use activates drug-metabolizing enzymes, its use may transform a drug into a toxic substance that can harm organs such as the liver. Drugs can also slow alcohol metabolism and result in a greater level of intoxication.

Alcohol and drug interactions may be affected by these other factors:

Among the elderly, the breakdown of chemicals in the liver, and their removal from the body by the kidneys, is greatly slowed. In addition, elderly individuals are often using multiple medications. Adding alcohol to this mix can quickly cause an unwanted interaction.

Fatigue and stress, as well as other health variables, may cause alcohol and drugs to interact, causing problem conditions.

Drug-elimination times affect its combination with alcohol. An example is the sedative and sleep aid Dalmane. A person may ingest 5 milligrams of Dalmane to get to sleep, and the next day, feeling fresh and having lunch at work, has a single beer and feels uncommonly drowsy because there is still Dalmane in his system but was not aware of that until he had the beer.

The route of administration of a drug can determine both the intensity and the duration of its effect. The most powerful effect is achieved from a smokable drug, followed by intravenous injection; oral ingestion is the least powerful.

Drug-preparation methods affect alcohol-drug interactions. Concerns have been raised about the interference of alcohol with timed-released drug formulas, in particular where the coatings of the tiny pills can be damaged by alcohol. This process can dump the entire dose into the small intestine, raising blood levels of the drugs to dangerous levels. Research is under way to develop new coatings that are not affected by the presence of alcohol (Lennernäs, 2009).

Because of all the above factors, it is often impossible to predict drug-alcohol interactions and their level of severity.

ALCOHOL TAKEN TOGETHER WITH ILLICIT DRUGS

Alcohol and illicit drugs taken together have a variety of interactions: Alcohol, for example, increases the sedative and depressing effect of marijuana. It also has an antagonistic or blocking effect on stimulants, and people sometimes use it to come down from a cocaine or amphetamine high. However, the combination is potentially very dangerous because alcohol, as well as powerful stimulants, elevates blood pressure, increasing the risk for heart attack and stroke. In addition, individuals binging on stimulants often experience paranoid thinking and aggressive motives. Adding alcohol, which impairs judgment and disinhibits behavior and emotion, increases the possibility of interpersonal violence, road rage, and other destructive behaviors. Alcohol also increases the sedative effect of opiate drugs such as heroin, and it depresses respiration. This result is common in many emergency-room visits and fatalities. (See Narcotics, below.)

ALCOHOL TAKEN TOGETHER WITH PRESCRIBED MEDICATIONS

The following information is about the effects of mixing alcohol and prescription medications, whether these medications were obtained legitimately or through theft or diversion. This information should not be used as the basis for making a decision on whether to combine alcohol with another drug or medication. Health care providers must be consulted in making this decision.

Antibiotics are used to fight infection. In combination with acute alcohol consumption, some antibiotics may cause nausea, vomiting, headache, and even seizures. Also, chronic alcohol use may decrease the effectiveness of antibiotics.

Anticoagulants (such as warfarin, sold under the brand name Coumadin) stop blood from clotting, which is a cause of stroke. Anticoagulant use increases the possibility of bleeding, and heavy drinking in combination with anticoagulants increases the risk of a fatal hemorrhage. Chronic alcoholism limits the benefits of anticoagulants.

Antidepressants are commonly prescribed medications in the United States. Because many people with depression self-medicate by drinking, this is a major risk area for alcohol-drug interaction. Alcohol increases the sedative effects of some antidepressants (especially tricyclics) and interferes with the ability of others to lift depressed moods. Red wine contains a chemical, tyramine, which can produce a dangerous spike in blood pressure for patients taking monoamine oxidase inhibitors (MAOIs), an older class of antidepressants.

Antidiabetic medications are medications that lower blood sugar (a hypoglycemic effect). Alcohol can interact with antidiabetic drugs to either lower or raise blood sugar and to produce nausea and headache.

Antihistamines are antiallergy medications commonly available without prescription. Many, such as diphenhydramine, marketed as Benadryl, cause sedation. Alcohol increases the sedative effects of antihistamines as well as dizziness.

Antipsychotic medications help diminish symptoms of psychosis such as hallucinations and delusions. Many of these medications produce a marked sedative effect that is increased by consumption of alcohol. Liver damage is also a risk in combining these substances.

Antiseizure medications used for seizure disorders such as epilepsy may be made more available in the bloodstream when drinking alcohol, raising the danger of side effects. However, in the chronic heavy drinker, the opposite may occur, and the drug is not as available to prevent seizures.

Cardiovascular (heart) medications are used to treat angina and high blood pressure. Acute alcohol consumption interacts with some of these drugs, causing dizziness or fainting when standing up (postural hypotension).

Narcotic pain relievers (i.e., opioid analgesics) are powerful. They are legitimately prescribed for postoperative pain, cancer pain, exposed dental nerves, and other moderate and severe pain. These include oxycodone (Oxycontin); many varieties of codeine combined with acetominophen, aspirin, or ibuprofen; meperidine (Demerol); and hydrocodone (Percocet). Combining a narcotic with alcohol has an additive or multiplying effect on these sedative substances, potentially leading to respiratory depression, coma, and death. Many emergency-room visits are the effect of narcotic-alcohol combinations. In addition, opiates slow gastric emptying, leading to higher concentrations of alcohol in the stomach.

Nonnarcotic pain relievers, including aspirin and ibuprofen, can contribute to stomach bleeding and failure of the blood to clot properly. Alcohol raises those risks. Continued heavy drinking can greatly raise the risk of liver damage from acetaminophen.

Opiate substitution therapies often use methadone. The sedative effect of methadone is enhanced by consumption of alcohol.

Sedatives and hypnotics are widely prescribed to reduce anxiety and as sleep aids. Most, such as diazepam (Valium) and clonazepam (Klonopin), are in the benzodiazepine class. Use of these medications with alcohol greatly enhances sedation and sleep, and many driving fatalities are a result of combining these substances. Lorazepam (Ativan), combined with alcohol, causes respiratory depression and lowered heart rate. The older class of sedatives, barbiturates, has been largely discontinued due to the small window of safety between a dose that works and a dose that kills. Combining alcohol with barbiturates is a recipe for disaster and was implicated in the death of Marilyn Monroe (Weathermon & Crabb, 1999).

ALCOHOL AND CAFFEINE

Caffeine masks some of the symptoms of alcohol intoxication. It can result in a wide-awake drunk who is not aware of his or her impaired motor skills, posing a menace if the person operates a vehicle. Moreover, he or she may end up with a higher blood alcohol level than would be probable if he or she were not under the influence of this stimulant, raising the probability of a blackout or alcohol poisoning.

Alcohol and caffeine are taken together in at least three ways: to sober up or stay awake, by consuming an energy drink such as Red Bull along with hard liquor, and by consuming manufactured beverages that contain alcohol and caffeine.

Combining Red Bull or a similar beverage and hard liquor, which allows the drinker to be intoxicated without being tired, has been popular for a few years among young adults wishing to party and/or dance all night in club settings. In addition to simply drinking an energy drink alternatively with hard liquors, bar patrons can order special cocktails, called Vod Bomb or DVR (double-vodka Red Bull).

In 2010, a scare concerning popular caffeinated and flavored malt beverages, including Four Loko and Joose, occurred when a number of college students who had consumed multiple cans of the beverages ended up in emergency rooms with alcohol poisoning. These drinks originally contained 12 percent alcohol, the same as wine, in a large can, thus providing the equivalent of from two to four standard drinks, as well as the amount of caffeine in one or two cups of coffee. In November 2010, in response to an anticipated governmental crackdown, the manufacturer of Four Loko voluntarily announced that it was taking caffeine out of the product. As several states moved to ban these beverages, on November 17, 2010, the Food and Drug Administration demanded that four manufacturers of canned malt beverages stop adding caffeine to their products. The equally dangerous Red Bull–vodka cocktails, however, have not been the focus of regulatory intervention.

CHAPTER 3

Key Terms and Definitions

All societies have ways of marking off which behaviors are considered reasonable and appropriate, and which are considered excessive or abnormal. These norms often include judgments about the proper amount of alcohol consumption, levels defined as excessive and problematic, and, especially in American culture, a level considered as indicating an addiction or a disease.

Definitions among laypersons tend to be more permissive than those in the professional health care and medical fields. As discussed in detail later in this volume, cultural concepts of illness, normality, and deviance affect classification schemes. For example, in a community where men sit on stoops and drink rum out of paper bags at 10 A.M., who is the alcohol abuser? As cultural attitudes toward alcoholism and other syndromes change, these may evolve into official categories. Cynics point out, however, that alcohol abusers are whoever we say they are, or whoever drinks more than we do.

The following section presents the two major professional systems of classification in the United States: those of the National Council on Alcoholism and Drug Dependence and of the latest edition of the American Psychiatric Association's diagnostic manual, informally known in the medical field as DSM-IV-TR. It also reflects changes to the manual proposed to take effect in 2013 with the publication of the fifth edition.

DEFINITIONS BY THE NATIONAL COUNCIL ON ALCOHOLISM AND DRUG DEPENDENCE

The National Council on Alcoholism and Drug Dependence (NCADD), originally the National Council on Alcoholism, which was influenced by the philosophy of Alcoholics Anonymous in its founding years, refined its longstanding definition of alcoholism in 1990. In addition, its definition was accepted by the American Society for Addiction Medicine. According to the NCADD, alcoholism is a primary chronic disease with genetic, psychosocial, and environmental factors influencing its development and manifestations. The disease is often progressive and fatal. It is characterized by continuous or periodic impaired control over drinking, preoccupation with alcohol, use of alcohol despite adverse consequences, and distortions in thinking, most notably denial. Within this definition, *primary* refers to the nature of alcoholism as a disease entity in addition to and separate from other pathophysiologic states that may be associated with it. The term suggests that alcoholism, as an addiction, is not a symptom of an underlying disease state (National Council on Alcoholism and Drug Dependence, 1990).

According to this definition, a drunkard has a disease, one that exists in its own right and is not, say, a symptom of depression. Furthermore, it is a disease with certain distinct and special characteristics: It is a chronic disease (persistent and reoccurring, such as are cancer and diabetes) rather than an acute illness (sudden and short term, such as strep throat). It is progressive (gets worse and worse), and it is tied in to certain thinking patterns that constitute a system of denial. This is the so-called American disease concept of alcoholism, originally described by E. M. Jellinek (1960) and updated by the NCADD in 1990, that is further discussed in this volume.

DSM-IV-TR DEFINITIONS

The official medical definitions of alcohol-use syndromes appear in a section in the bible of psychiatry, the *Diagnostic and Statistical Manual of Mental Disorders*, fourth edition, text revision, or DSM-IV-TR (American Psychological Association, 2000), along with other substance-use disorders and, of course, a whole range of disorders from dyslexia to schizophrenia. The DSM-IV-TR has made an important distinction between alcohol dependence (alcoholism or alcohol addiction) and alcohol abuse—a less pernicious condition. Also, in the DSM-IV-TR criteria for alcohol dependence, there is no mention of disease progression or denial. The following section consists of an edited version of the DSM-IV-TR criteria for diagnosing alcohol dependence and alcohol abuse.

Alcohol Dependence—Diagnostic Code 303.90

Alcohol use leading to significant impairment or distress. Three or more of the following conditions occur in the same 12-month period:

- Tolerance is a need to drink much more alcohol to become intoxicated or achieve another desired effect such as stress reduction or sleep. If the alcoholic uses only the same amount, the effect is minimal.

- Withdrawal syndrome occurs when alcohol use is stopped or even reduced. Alcoholics must drink to avoid these symptoms, collectively known as the shakes.
- Alcohol is often used in larger amounts or over a longer period than was intended.
- Unsuccessful efforts are undertaken to cut down or control alcohol use.
- A great deal of time is spent in activities necessary to obtain or use alcohol or to recover from its effects.
- Normal activities are given up or reduced because of alcohol use.
- Alcohol use is continued despite knowledge of having a persistent physical or psychological problem likely to have been caused or exacerbated by alcohol (as, an alcohol-related ulcer).

A full-fledged physical addiction need not be present for a person to receive the diagnosis of alcohol dependence. In fact, the vast majority of those classified as alcoholic do not have physical dependence, although they may be psychologically dependent.

Alcohol Abuse—Diagnostic Code 305.00

Alcohol use leading to significant impairment or distress. One (or more) of the following conditions occur within a 12-month period:

- Alcohol use results in a failure to fulfill major role obligations at work, school, or home (e.g., absenteeism, poor performance, child neglect).
- Alcohol use occurs in situations in which it is physically hazardous (e.g., drunk driving).
- Alcohol-related legal problems (e.g., arrests for alcohol-related disorderly conduct) occur.
- Continued alcohol abuse occurs despite the presence of social or interpersonal problems caused or exacerbated by the effects of the alcohol (e.g., arguments or fights).

A person in this category has never met the criteria for alcohol dependence.

In a discussion area, the DSM-IV-TR also distinguishes between abuse and "nonpathological substance use (e.g., social drinking)" (American Psychological Association, 2000, p. 207). There are also alcohol-related conditions, including the one described in the manual's section titled "303.00 Alcohol Intoxication" (pp. 214–215). That is, a person may be seriously drunk but may not receive a diagnosis of alcohol abuse or dependence because he or she may be experimenting with alcohol or may even have been forced to drink excessively, such as in a hazing ritual. There is no scale to tell us how many episodes of severe intoxication will trigger the diagnosis of alcohol abuse or dependence.

Application of diagnostic criteria toward the making of a diagnosis requires interviewing skills and a judgment call by health care providers (Yalisove, 2004, p. 35). For example, exactly how many bouts of intoxication have occurred? Can we trust the responses of the patient to questions as he or she faces being forced into treatment? Are our interviewing techniques making the client minimize his or her drinking or clam up altogether?

DSM-5 DEFINITIONS

Proposed revisions to the DSM system (American Psychological Association, 2010a, 2010b) to be included in the fifth edition, known informally as DSM-5 (the use of roman numerals to designate the edition is being discontinued) are in preparation and include combining alcohol dependence and alcohol abuse into a single category called alcohol-use disorder.

The rationale is as follows: First, for a diagnosis to be considered a reliable category, patients, on reexamination, should come up with the same diagnosis. Studies (see Hasin & Besler, 1999; Hasin, Paykin, Endicott, & Grant, 2009) show that while the alcohol-dependence category is reliable, the alcohol-abuse category was not; on reexamination, patients come and go from that category. Second, the most common way for alcohol abuse to be diagnosed is with a single criterion such as drunk driving. The framers of DSM-5 call into question this approach, which does not necessarily warrant a psychiatric diagnosis. Finally, because of the considerable gray area between the abuse category or the dependence category, it is unclear whether persons fit into one or the other.

The new category will resemble the DSM-IV-TR's definition of alcohol dependence, with moderate severity indicated if two or more criteria are met and an indication of severe severity called for if four or more criteria are met. The presence of craving will also be added as a criterion for diagnosis if the proposals are finalized.

CHAPTER 4

Risk Factors for Alcohol Misuse and Worsening of Abuse

RISK FACTORS

Millions of young people experiment with alcohol without progression into alcohol abuse, and millions of adult citizens drink responsibly and moderately. Yet for some, use creates minor, moderate, or even fatal problems. Factors that propel alcohol experimentation into to alcohol misuse or abuse exist at many levels, ranging from molecular and genetic strata to individual personality development, family and community parameters, and broad social and cultural considerations. The mixture of risk factors will be unique to every individual who have developed alcohol use disorders.

Alcohol and Genetics: Risk Factors Rooted in Inherited Characteristics

The study of genetic risk factors for alcohol-use disorders is still tentative and subject to much debate (Buckland, 2008). Individuals at risk for alcohol-use disorders probably have inherited more than one risk factor (Nurnberger & Bierut, 2007; Reich, Hinrichs, Culverhouse, & Bierut, 1999), including but not limited to those predisposing for various psychiatric disorders. Ducci and Goldman (2008) estimate that approximately half of the liability for alcohol use is genetic, although few others credit genetics with such great influence. Complex behaviors (like getting off the couch and going down to the liquor store) are not inherited, but some specific characteristic of how the nervous system operates, or how a chemical is metabolized, are.

In children of alcoholics, the rate at which alcohol is metabolized decreases after a first so-called primer drink. Such individuals will have to drink more to obtain the desired effect, and are at risk for alcohol abuse (Bradford, Karnitsching, Powell, & Garbutt, 2007; Schuckit, 2009).

Children of alcoholics exhibit more sensitization to alcohol as blood-alcohol level rises and more tolerance as blood-alcohol level falls. Alcohol is more rewarding because the pleasurable, excitatory aspects of initial intoxication is increased (in other words, they get drunk easily), and the feelings of anxiety and depression that can come on as blood-alcohol levels drop are reduced compared to children of nonalcoholics (Newlin & Thomson, 1990).

Increasingly, antisocial-personality disorder (sociopathy) is seen as having a biological basis: Sociopaths' physiological responses and brain-wave activity are different from that of normals. People with antisocial-personality disorder are frequently heavy drinkers and substance abusers (Dick & Agrawal, 2008). A genetic substrate for impulsivity, sensation seeking, and behavioral disinhibition, a temperament that can be a feature of antisocial personality, is associated with alcohol-use disorders (Schuckit, 2009).

Individuals who experience difficulty in screening out stimuli, which causes them to feel overwhelmed, may lead them to self-medicate. Differences in the ability to screen out stimuli have genetic roots, and this problem occurs especially in families and/or cultures that drink a lot.

A biological and genetic substrate exists for severe problems regulating moods, such as getting easily upset and having difficulty in coming back to a baseline, or normal, mood, which occurs in the cases of people with borderline personality disorder (Skodol et al., 2002), who are greatly at risk for alcoholism (Myers, 2008).

Having a relative with schizophrenia is a risk factor for alcohol-use disorders, aside from the stress of living in a family with mental illness (Smith, Barch, Wolf, Mamah, & Csernansky, 2008). These individuals have inherited a neurological vulnerability that is not yet entirely understood.

Hyperactive temperament, indicated by difficulty in being calm, sleeping, and relaxing, and in having attentional difficulties (ADHD), leads to self-medication. Children of alcoholics have higher rates of ADHD (Earls, Reich, Jung, & Cloninger, 1988).

Other risk factors at the genetic and biological level include having intrusive thoughts, as in obsessive-compulsive disorder, suffering from pervasive anxiety, and inherited depressive disorders or other mood disorders, including bipolar disorder. Some researchers (Gorwood, Bellivier,

Adès, & Leboyer, 2000) believe that populations of persons with bipolar disorder, and of alcoholics, share the DR D2 gene.

From time to time, researchers claim to find a genetic magic bullet: a gene linked to alcoholism. Oversimplified accounts find their way into newsmagazines and onto numerous Web sites, and even into textbooks, as a new so-called alcoholic gene is proclaimed. Readers should be skeptical about these discoveries: First, the influence of a gene is not directly on human behavior. Genes determine responses on the level of what amino acids will configure within a protein or at what rate a neurotransmitter substance breaks down. They cannot get someone off the couch, down the elevator, and off to the liquor store to buy a pint of 100-proof Southern Comfort; there are countless intervening variables. The risk factors at different levels also exhibit a great deal of interplay. Take, for example, a young person with attention-deficit hyperactivity disorder. Alcohol abusers number within their ranks a disproportionate number of people with ADHD (Molina & Pelham, 2003; Smith, Molina, & Pelham, 2002). Their drinking may reflect not only difficulties in sleeping and calming down but also the fact that their parents also suffered from ADHD and provided a chaotic and inconsistent home environment, and that they enrolled in a school where they were stigmatized and ostracized for their behavior—so-called environmental blowback—not to mention the existence of drinking subcultures toward which they can gravitate. In addition, a single gene, depending on myriad factors, may or may not be activated. We may find it in a genetic screen, but it may lay dormant, as in the case of a carrier of sickle-cell anemia.

Studies claiming to find alcoholic genes are popularized in the press as great breakthroughs before often quickly falling by the wayside. A cautionary example is the discovery of a supposed alcoholic gene popularized by Dr. Kenneth Blum. According to Blum's research, alcoholics, other substance abusers, and even individuals who compulsively gamble or engage in sex are more likely to have a gene that renders them unable to achieve pleasure from stimuli as normal individuals do. He dubbed this condition the reward-deficiency syndrome (Blum & Payne, 1991; Blum et al., 2008). This research caught on in the recovery community and was widely quoted in the popular press and across the Internet. Critics of this hypothesis (Peele, 1992), however, state that though such a condition could exist, this single gene cannot be given so much credit for causing addiction.

Subsequent research (Gelernter, Goldman, & Risch, 1993) did not replicate the original findings that the so-called Blum gene is found more often in alcoholics.

Alcohol and Personality Development

Personality is broadly defined as the individual organization of emotional and behavioral patterns into a self during the psychosocial developmental process.

There is no one alcoholic personality. However, problems that arise as individuals learn to organize their emotions, behavior, and attitudes into a coherent self may in turn affect their use of psychoactive substances, especially alcohol. Risk factors at the level of personality development and individual thinking patterns may include depression, resistance to trust, experience with trauma, and unresolved grief and loss.

Learned helplessness and hopelessness in thinking and behavior leads to depression. This conclusion is based on the famous experiments of Martin Seligman in 1965 in which dogs were placed in an enclosure from which they could not escape. They were given warning that a mild shock was about to be administered. After some attempts to escape, they gave up and sat whining. Next, walls preventing their escape to a neighboring enclosure were removed, and they had the ability to escape the shocks. However, they continued to sit and cry rather than jump off the electrified platform. Seligman (1975) made this experiment into a model of human depression, concluding that people who had learned or been taught that they were helpless and hopeless would not actively pursue their goals or have a fulfilling life, and would experience depression. According to Seligman, their depression was rooted in maladaptive cognition and behavior. Closely related to depression is low self-esteem—or negative self schemas and self-concept disturbances, as researchers variously refer to it—were found to be major risk factors for alcohol abuse (Corte & Zucker, 2008).

Substance abusers often have difficulty in developing trust, and a sense of safety and consistency in the environment. Having a parent with ADHD can be a risk factor for this experience (Marshal, Molina, Pelham, & Cheong, 2007). Having a parent with a substance-abuse disorder is likely to influence development of social phobia and anxiety disorders that will lead to self-medication (Pagano et al., 2007).

Experience of trauma, and expectation of punishment, attack, or catastrophe, lead to self-medication (Widom & Hiller-Sturmhofel, 2001). A large percentage of veterans treated in the U.S. Department of Veterans Affairs system for alcoholism have a co-occurring condition of posttraumatic stress disorder (Boudewyns, Woods, Hyer, & Albrecht, 1991; Hoge et al., 2004).

Unresolved grief and loss, which can result from loss of family and friends, a shift in body image, or a loss of identity based on a change in employment or other form of affiliation, prompts self-medication. Thus, retirement among white males in America is a risk factor.

Risk Factors at the Level of the Family and Peer Group

Risks in the family and peer environment include heavy drinking in the family and peer group, the use of alcohol to deal with anger, boredom in the family and peer group, abusive and inconsistent parenting, chaotic home environment, and domestic and sexual abuse (Widom & Hiller-Sturmhofel, 2001). Other risks are tolerance of alcohol-related problematic behaviors in the family and peer group, peer pressure for use, peer norms encouraging alcohol misuse, and inaccurate estimation of peer norms for use and peer level of use (Perkins & Craig, 2003).

Students in grades 7–12 whose parents utilized an authoritative parental style marked by firm, consistent, engaged behavior, as opposed to authoritarian, neglectful, or indulgent styles, were less likely to engage in heavy drinking or have friends who drank heavily (Bahr & Hoffmann, 2010).

Risk Factors at the Level of the Community

Some characteristics of communities that constitute risk factors for alcohol abuse include powerful alcohol-abuse subcultures and traditions such as so-called frontloading at sports events, in which participants drink heavily before entering the venue; as well as the absence of alternative activities to drinking alcohol. Other risk factors are availability as seen in the prevalence of liquor stores and bars in certain neighborhoods, the lack of a stable community support system (and the prevalence of community disorganization in general), economic stressors in housing and employment, the presence of gang activity in a community, and lack of attachment to school by students and parents (Hawkins, Catalano, & Arthur, 2002; Hawkins, Catalano & Miller, 1992; Hawkins, Lishner, Catalano, & Howard, 1986).

Risk Factors in the Broader Society and Culture

Blame it on the goose, gotcha feeling loose (Grey Goose vodka)
Blame it on the 'tron, catch me in a zone (Patron tequila)
                    Excerpt from Jamie Foxx rap video (Brown et al., 2009)

The broader sociocultural environment provides many risk factors for misuse of alcohol, including exposure to alcohol advertising in general and in association with sports events and the targeting of age and/or ethnic groups by alcoholic-beverage interests. Solitary and same-sex drinking are risk factors in cultures worldwide.

American culture identifies alcohol as sophisticated, adult, sexy, something that facilitates socializing and sex, and a tension reducer. The culture also identifies the beginning of alcohol use as a rite of passage.

Alcohol use is a theme in music. An analysis of the 297 most popular songs of 2005 found that about three-fourths of rap songs and about one-third of country-western songs portrayed substance use (Primack et al., 2008); note the excerpted lyrics from a rap video referenced above, which also associates alcohol with the availability of sex. Other studies have found that the drinking theme in country-western music is both romanticized and associated with negative consequences, failure, loneliness, and lost love (Chalfont & Beckley, 1977; Conners & Alpher, 1998). Furthermore, depressive and alcoholic themes in that music genre are actually associated with higher rates of suicide among working-class whites with preexisting proneness to commit suicide (Gundlach, 1992).

The latter conclusion exemplifies the combination of risk factors at different levels, in this case a subcultural context of hard-drinking white country-music fans within which a predilection toward suicide may be present for any number of reasons. Another example is the presence of physical pain due to accidents or illness in a rural cultural context that scorns the use of pain medication and underutilizes medical intervention but uses whiskey as an analgesic and sedative (Jennings, 2010).

WORSENING OF ABUSE: THE VICIOUS CYCLES

Few people are immune to all the risk factors mentioned above, and few are immune to financial and social stressors in modern life, which can be crushing. Many people who have experimented or have drank responsibly may begin to do so maladaptively, neglecting responsibilities and experiencing negative consequences such as a suspended driver's license, drunk-and-disorderly convictions, and sanctions at work. Thus, they meet the criteria for alcohol abuse according to the DSM-IV-TR.

At this level, various vicious cycles kick in and the syndrome tends to worsen. At the same time, motives and pressures toward normalcy present themselves, and coercion, or periodic attempts to rein in, reverse, or stabilize the slide toward severe abuse and alcoholism, may occur.

Several vicious cycles facilitate the progression of alcohol abuse in the direction of alcohol dependence and interlock with one another to form a perfect storm. There is the development of metabolic tolerance, which leads the abuser to drink more to feel normal, as well as an increase in behavioral tolerance that masks high blood-alcohol levels. Cerebral functioning, which includes perception and judgment, memory, organization and consistency, and impulse control, is impaired, and alcoholic blackouts may occur. These impairments lead to negative social and economic consequences and a sense of loss of control. In addition, negative social consequences of alcohol abuse, such as legal, financial, family, and occupational difficulties, generate emotional pain and a sense of helplessness and failure.

On top of all this, stigmatizing labels applied to the abuser contribute to low self-esteem, hopelessness, and the internalization and acceptance of identity as an alcohol abuser, a failure, and a deviant. The drinker suffers ostracism and isolation, and may tend to gravitate toward networks and subcultures of alcohol abusers that reward and validate drinking patterns. The negative physical and medical consequences of alcohol misuse cause physical and emotional pain and deterioration that can be masked by self-medicating.

As is chronicled in many self-help works, family members, peers, and social networks are responsible for considerable enabling of abuse. Examples include bailing an arrested abuser out of jail, calling in excuses, and providing financial support while self-destructive behavior is taking place so that the abuser can spiral down without a reality check, buffered against facing the realities and consequences of the abuse that might provide a rude awakening. One extreme example is that of two sisters who sought out their alcoholic brother, who often ended up passing out on the street. They routinely carried him home, undressed him and bathed off his vomit and urine, and put him to bed. The abuser and his family, peers, and colleagues may not only enable abuse but also deny, minimize, and rationalize alcohol misuse and alcohol-related problem behaviors. Abuse may nestle in a workplace culture of drinking where supervisors are former peers; members of the organization who are embarrassed to intervene participate in organizational denial.

CHAPTER 5

Phases and Stages of Alcoholism: Theoretical Considerations

The definition of extremely heavy problem drinking as a special disease called alcoholism is a particularly American invention, and one that emerged from self-help movements to dominate public health and clinical practice. The evolution of this concept is explored in this section, and its attempt to outline the stages in the development of alternative models is presented toward the end of the section.

ELVIN MORTON JELLINEK: PHASES

Although Benjamin Rush described alcoholism as a disease in 1784, and the temperance movement in the 19th century recognized alcoholism as an addictive phenomenon, a scientific elaboration of the concept didn't take hold until the mid 20th century. E. M. Jellinek (1890–1963), a biostatistician by training, is perhaps the best-known theorist on alcoholism. Jellinek's initial 1946 study of alcohol as a disease, based on a self-reporting questionnaire by AA members, was funded by Marty Mann, one of the first female members of Alcoholics Anonymous (if not the first) and founder of the AA-backed National Council on Alcoholism, and by R. Brinkley Smithers, a philanthropist who supported alcoholism programs (Jellinek, 1946). He elaborated this research into what he called the disease concept of alcoholism and, as such, founded the paradigm that become dominant in addiction treatment (Jellinek, 1960). Jellinek was the scientific face of the Alcoholics Anonymous recovery movement, and his message resonated greatly with that organization. In his tabulation of what the AA members reported on their worsening condition, he produced a framework to describe the progression of alcoholic disease.

Prealcoholic Phase

In this phase, which lasts several months to several years, the individual is not yet an abuser, but the groundwork is being laid. A prealcoholic

- is socially motivated to use alcohol.
- experiences psychological relief as a result of drinking.
- learns to seek out drinking situations.
- develops a growth in metabolic tolerance to alcohol.

Prodromal (Presyndrome) Phase

In this phase, Jellinek says, many warning signs of impending alcoholism are manifesting themselves. People in this phrase certainly are alcohol abusers as defined in the DSM-IV-TR, and fairly severe ones at that. Prodromal drinkers

- drink more heavily than their peers.
- are habitually drunk.
- experience blackouts (temporary amnesia).
- gulp and sneak drinks and drink before parties.
- feel guilty about their behavior and avoid discussion of drinking.
- suffer chronic hangovers.

Crucial Phase

In this phase, the individual is really becoming alcohol dependent or alcoholic. Drinkers in the crucial phase

- develop elaborate systems of alibis, excuses, and reasons for their drinking.
- indulge in eye openers, or morning drinking.
- make futile attempts to stop drinking.
- drink alone or with other alcoholics.
- brood over imagined wrongs and are paranoid.
- experience loss of family, friends, and employment.
- seek medical attention but don't comply with instructions.

Chronic Phase (or Severe Alcoholism)

Chronic drinkers

- go on benders, during which they remain drunk for days.
- disregard all responsibilities.
- suffer serious acute withdrawal syndrome, including tremors and hallucinations.
- protect their supply of alcohol carefully.
- are plagued by resentments, fears, and anxieties.
- experience a collapse of their system of alibis.
- are at risk of death from cirrhosis of the liver or another alcohol-related syndrome.

TYPES OF ALCOHOLISM: JELLINEK'S SPECIES

Over the next 12 years, Jellinek recognized that there are different alcoholisms. He named these as species, as if they were categories of creature. Although species are not often used in practice nowadays, they are of historical interest as an attempt to come to grips with the important variations in alcohol-use syndromes. The species are named after Greek letters:

- An Alpha alcoholic has a purely psychological dependence on alcohol. There is no loss of control and no inability to abstain, but the drinker relies on alcohol to remediate problems and stresses in life. This problem drinker may or may not progress to later stages.
- A Beta alcoholic has physical problems but is not physically or psychologically dependent. Betas crop up in heavy-drinking cultures with inadequate nutrition, such as Russia.
- A Gamma alcoholic is a severe, physically and psychologically dependent, out-of-control alcoholic. The sample of alcoholics sampled by Jellinek in constructing his disease theory were Gammas and were typical of early Alcoholics Anonymous members.
- A Delta alcoholic is almost like a Gamma, but without loss of control. A Delta goes to work but keeps a bottle of whiskey in a drawer, and cannot abstain even for one day.
- An Epsilon alcoholic is a periodic or binge drinker, as opposed to a relapsing Gamma.

Jellinek was not sure whether Alphas or Epsilons were true bearers of alcoholic disease or whether their drinking was symptomatic of other problems.

Later in this volume, there is a description of the controversy over the term "binge drinking."

STAGES OF ALCOHOLISM ACCORDING TO VERNON JOHNSON

Episcopal priest Vernon Johnson was a recovering alcoholic who made two important contributions to the alcoholism field. He is probably best known for formulating the formal intervention process to force alcoholics into treatment. His book *I'll Quit Tomorrow* (Johnson, 1973) has gone through seven editions, plus five addition editions as *Intervention* (Johnson, 1986). In his works, he also presents a model for the progression of alcoholism, largely centering around moods and mood swings, which lie on a simple line with three components: pain, normal, and euphoria. Johnson spelled out the emotional ramifications of disease progression on 12 charts, which have been considerably boiled down in the following description:

Pain			Normal		Euphoria		
−4	−3	−2	−1	1	2	3	4

In Phase I, drinkers learn that a drink moves them from a normal to a pleasant mood and back again to normal, from 1 to 2 and back to 1. They then learn that the degree of a mood swing is controlled by the dosage ingested, so that they may go up to 3 and back to 1.

In Phase II, drinkers seek out the mood swing and drink excessively at times but have no real emotional costs associated with doing so as yet, going from 1 to 4 and back.

In Phase III, the beginning of harmful dependence, drinkers slips down below 1 after drinking into a painful place, as with experiencing a hangover, guilt, and depression. They are uncomfortable about their level of drinking and its emotional cost, and they are starting to feel overwhelmed, raising some unconscious defenses (Johnson, 1973, p. 17). During this phase, the backswing takes them all the way down to a minus 3 or 4. Their self-image has waned considerably as their drunken behavior has had consequences. In the final subphase of Phase III, drinkers have suicidal tendencies, and they have locked in a free-floating mass of negative feelings, papered over by rationalizations and defenses. This is Johnson's description of what he dubs "alcoholic depression."

In Phase IV, drinkers are chronically depressed and have to drink to feel normal. However, they end up feeling even worse. This phase can be charted as moving from a minus 3 to minus 1 and down to minus 4.

MODELS OF ALCOHOLISM

A model is a description of an object or phenomenon. It can be constructed with glue and strips of wood, as with a model airplane, with pictures, or with ideas. In the social sciences, models are theories that present the essentials of personal and social behavior, and they may attempt an explanation. Models for alcoholism include the moral model, the temperance model, the American disease model, the religious model, the characterological model, the conditional or behavioral model, the biological model, and the general-systems model.

The moral model emphasizes deficits in personal responsibility or spiritual strength as the root of alcohol abuse and alcoholism. This model was mainly associated with a religious, 19th-century viewpoint, but it persists today. For example, drunk driving, an act of willful misconduct, is a crime whether the individual is diagnosed as alcoholic or not. Many citizens still view alcoholics as moral failures.

The temperance model, developed in the mid-19th century, saw alcohol as a dangerous drug that led to ruination. This philosophy led to the Prohibition era (1919–1933). Antialcohol messages of today still have a tone that rings of crusading temperance activism, although perhaps without taking an ax to casks of whiskey. Critics of the federal law that set the legal drinking age at 21 say that that restriction is an artifact of this model.

The American disease model stems from Alcoholics Anonymous, which came into being two years after the repeal of Prohibition. The crucial tenets of this model are that alcoholism is a progressive, irreversible condition characterized primarily by loss of control over drinking. According to the model, alcoholism cannot be cured, only arrested by complete abstinence. In early AA literature and meetings, alcoholics were said to be different constitutionally from nonalcoholics, which makes it impossible for them to drink moderately or without problems except for during rare, short periods. As described in detail in the first part of this section, pioneering alcoholism researcher Elton Morton Jellinek put a scientific stamp on the disease model.

In Alcoholics Anonymous, denial is a central feature of alcoholism (Alcoholics Anonymous, 1976). The disease model, as explained within AA, also has a spiritual component. Alcoholism is seen not only as a physical and psychological disease but also as a spiritual one, and recovery from alcoholism has a crucial spiritual aspect.

Religious or purely spiritual models, often considered folk models because they derive from the rank-and-file citizenry, are found in several faiths. As described in the section on culture and drugs, women in New York's South Bronx neighborhood described to one of the authors how spirits or demons were responsible for their husbands' heavy drinking.

According to the characterological view, deficiencies in personality functioning and mental pathology cause alcohol abuse. This model was originally rooted in Freudian psychoanalysis, which addressed alcoholism in the era after World War II. Alcoholics were said to be fixated at the oral stage or to suffer from latent homosexuality, or were subject to other classic psychoanalytic interpretations. Some early addiction treatment considered the addict to have a character or personality disorder hidden behind a double wall of encapsulation created by emotional withdrawal and chemical anesthesia (Myers & Salt, 2007).

In the conditioning, or behaviorist, model, excessive drinking is seen as a pattern of learned behavior that has been reinforced. This interpretation lingers in some current treatment approaches such as community reinforcement, and incentives for attending treatment. In general, behaviorism is now meshed with cognitive approaches in most modern evidenced-based treatments.

The biological model credits inherited genetic and physiological factors as described in biological psychiatry and psychopharmacology, as were outlined in the previous section on risk factors, such as inherited attention-deficit hyperactivity disorder, depression, or inability to screen out stressful stimuli.

The general-systems model takes the social systems surrounding the alcoholic as crucial, most often the family. The family, like all systems, needs to maintain the status quo; therefore, without family treatment, the recovery quest is doomed.

The modern addiction field recognizes that all system levels are involved with alcoholism. It is a physical, psychosocial, family, community, and societal issue.

CHAPTER 6

Alcohol and Social Problems

Alcohol consumption has occurred for up to ten thousand years. Although much or most of that consumption has consisted of normal nutritional or recreational use, over that time, it has been a leading cause of mortality and disability. It is also linked to crime, violence, property, and law-enforcement costs, marital breakdown, and major losses in industrial productivity (Chisholm et al., 2004). Even so, the definition of heavy alcohol use as a social problem is a social and cultural construction and not a scientific fact like the existence of electrons and protons.

COST OF ALCOHOL TO SOCIETY

According to the World Health Organization (2010a),

Many of the varied health effects have been discovered fairly recently. Alcohol consumption has health and social consequences via intoxication (drunkenness), dependence (habitual, compulsive, and long-term drinking), and other biochemical effects. In addition to chronic diseases that may affect drinkers after many years of heavy use, alcohol contributes to traumatic outcomes that kill or disable at a relatively young age, resulting in the loss of many years of life to death or disability. There is increasing evidence that besides volume of alcohol, the pattern of the drinking is relevant for the health outcomes. Overall, there is a causal relationship between alcohol consumption and more than 60 types of disease and injury. Alcohol is estimated to cause about 20–30% worldwide of esophageal cancer, liver cancer, cirrhosis of the liver, homicide, epilepsy, and motor vehicle accidents.... Worldwide, alcohol causes 1.8 million deaths (3.2% of total) and [4% of the disability]. Unintentional injuries alone account for about one-third of the 1.8 million deaths, while neuropsychiatric conditions account for close to 40% of the 58.3 million deaths.

In the United States, alcohol is the most widely used drug: Over 8 percent of employed adult workers and almost 11 percent of adults with Medicaid or no health insurance either abuse or are dependent on alcohol. In 2005, the economic costs were estimated to have been $220 billion (27% direct, 73% indirect), with an average 3.8 percent annual increase. The health care costs from alcohol-related problems amount to more than $26 billion annually. That's $686 for every person living in the United States (Marin Institute, 2009).

The major factors related to alcohol abuse that are linked to economic costs (in order) are (1) lost productivity due to morbidity (i.e., illness and disease), (2) lost future earnings due to premature deaths, including motor vehicle crashes and other alcohol-related causes, (3) medical consequences of alcohol consumption, including fetal alcohol syndrome, (4) lost earnings due to crime, including those incarcerated, and (5) effects of the criminal justice system that address violent offenses, property damage and theft, and other alcohol-defined offenses. Other issues related to cost are treatment and prevention services, research, training, fire destruction and property damage, and social insurance (National Institute on Alcohol Abuse and Alcoholism, 2002). Motor vehicle–related injuries are the leading cause of death for people ages 1–34, and each year, nearly 5 million people sustain injuries stemming from alcohol abuse that require a visit to a hospital emergency department. The economic impact is also notable: Motor vehicle crashes cost around $230 billion in 2000 (Centers for Disease Control and Prevention, 2009; Substance Abuse and Mental Health Services Administration, 2009).

For youth, according to the Pacific Institute for Research and Evaluation, "underage drinking cost the citizens of the United States $68 billion in 2007. These costs include medical care, work loss, and pain and suffering associated with the multiple problems resulting from the use of alcohol.... Excluding pain and suffering from these costs, the direct costs of underage drinking incurred through medical care and loss of work cost the United States $22.3 billion each year" (Pacific Institute for Research and Evaluation, 2009). (See table 6.1.)

Clearly, the cost of problem alcohol use is considerable; however, some people claim that the government amount is "preposterously inflated[, failing] to balance the economic costs with the economic benefit [, including] the enormous contributions to the state and national economies and tax revenues from licensed beverages [and] jobs...involved" (Ford, 2010).

From Europe, it has been reported that the social costs of alcohol tend to be 1–3 percent of a given nation's gross national product (GDP), a basic measure of a country's overall economic output. For the European Union

Table 6.1 Costs of Underage Drinking by Problem in the United States, 2007

Problem	Total Costs (in millions)
Youth Violence	$43,835.8
Youth Traffic Crashes	$10,019.3
High-Risk Sex, Ages 14–20	$4,871.3
Youth Property Crime	$3,178.8
Youth Injury	$2,064.5
Poisonings and Psychoses	$416.2
Fetal Alcohol Spectrum Disorder among Mothers Age 15–20	$1,227.3
Youth Alcohol Treatment	$2,400.3
Total	**$68,001.5**

Source: Pacific Institute for Research and Evaluation (2009).

in 1998, the social costs of alcohol have been estimated at $65 billion–$195 billion at 1990 prices. According to the Institute of Alcohol Studies, "These figures are comparable to, or even exceed, government expenditures on social security and welfare, and approximate to 25 percent of health-service expenditure. The total value of the U.K. alcoholic-drinks market alone exceeds £30 billion, with sales of beer accounting for more than half of the amount" (Institute of Alcohol Studies, 2006).

Alcohol and Driving

According to the World Health Organization, auto-vehicle fatalities—many of them involving alcohol-impaired drivers—are one of the main causes of morbidity and mortality worldwide (Murray & Lopez, 1996). In 2008, in the United States, 11,773 people died in drunk-driving crashes involving a driver with an illegal blood-alcohol concentration (.08 or greater). These deaths constitute 31.6 percent of the 37,261 total traffic fatalities in 2008 (National Highway Traffic Safety Administration, 2009).

Alcohol-related crashes in the United States cost the public an estimated $114.3 billion in 2000 (Taylor et al., 2002). People other than a drinking driver paid $71.6 billion of the alcohol-related crash bill, which is 63 percent of the total cost of these crashes. These statistics come as no surprise when we consider that 15 percent of adults self-reported that they drove drunk in 2007. States with the highest rates of adults ages 18 or older driving within the last year while under the influence of alcohol among adults ages 18 or older were Wisconsin (26.4%), North Dakota (24.9%), Minnesota (23.5%), Nebraska (22.9%), and South Dakota (21.6%) (Office of Applied Studies, 2008). In the United States, annual alcohol-related

Table 6.2 Drunk Driving Fatalities

	Total Fatalities	Alcohol-Related Fatalities	
Year	Number	Number	Percent
1982	43,945	26,173	60
1983	42,589	24,635	58
1984	44,257	24,762	56
1985	43,825	23,167	53
1986	46,087	25,017	54
1987	46,390	24,094	52
1988	47,087	23,833	51
1989	45,582	22,424	49
1990	44,599	22,587	51
1991	41,508	20,159	49
1992	39,250	18,290	47
1993	40,150	17,908	45
1994	40,716	17,308	43
1995	41,817	17,732	42
1996	42,065	17,749	42
1997	42,013	16,711	40
1998	41,501	16,673	40
1999	41,717	16,572	40
2000	41,945	17,380	41
2001	42,196	17,400	41
2002	43,005	17,524	41
2003	42,643	17,013	40
2004	42,518	16,919	39
2005	43,443	16,885	39
2006	42,532	15,829	37
2007	41,059	15,387	37
2008	37,261	13,846	37

traffic fatalities have dropped by one-half in the past 25 years, from 26,000 to 13,000. (See table 6.2.) There is no other public-health victory that compares with this other than, perhaps, the fall in rates of smoking.

How drunk do you have to get to be a menace? Table 6.3 provides an overview. (Note: Flicker fusion is the frequency at which an intermittent light stimulus appears to be completely steady to the observer.)

According to this summary, the chances of a traffic accident are increased even at levels one-eighth to one-fourth the legally intoxicated level (0.01–0.019), where the driver may experience drowsiness and impaired

Table 6.3 Impairment of Drivers by Drinking Alcohol

BAC (g/dL)	By Lowest BAC at Which Impairment Was Found	By First BAC at Which 50% or More of Behavioral Tests Indicated Consistent Impairment
0.100	Critical Flicker Fusion	Simple Reaction Time, Critical Flicker Fusion
0.090–0.099		
0.080–0.089		
0.070–0.079		
0.060–0.069		Cognitive Tasks, Psychomotor Skills, Choice Reaction Time
0.050–0.059		Tracking
0.040–0.049	Simple Reaction Time	Perception, Visual Functions
0.030–0.039	Vigilance, Perception	Vigilance
0.020–0.029	Choice Reaction Time, Visual Functions	
0.010–0.019	Drowsiness, Psychomotor Skills, Cognitive Tasks, Tracking	Drowsiness
0.001–0.009	Driving, Flying, Divided Attention	Driving, Flying, Divided Attention

Source: National Highway Traffic Safety Administration (2000a).

psychomotor skills, cognition, and tracking ability. At blood-alcohol levels at or below the legal limit, a driver's reaction time may be reduced by up to 30 percent, vision may become blurred, and the judgment of distance, speed, and hazards is likely to be reduced. The diminished capacities of intoxicated drivers imperil themselves and others on the road; more so, heavy drinkers are less able to estimate their own sedation. They often do not recognize the cues that moderate drinkers do that they are in no shape to drive (Marczinski, Harrison, & Fillmore, 2008). Moreover, middle-class, moderately intoxicated individuals think that drunk-driving warnings are targeted at alcoholics or severely drunken persons, not at the person who has had a couple of drinks. The Advertising Council of America has come up with a campaign that declares, "Buzzed driving is drunk driving."

Here are some additional facts on drunk driving to consider: The risk of being killed in a single-vehicle crash is 11 times greater when blood-alcohol concentrations are between 0.05 and 0.09 percent than if there is no alcohol in the bloodstream (Zador, 1991). Studies have also shown that crashes involving alcohol are more likely to be fatal or to result in severe injuries (Moskowitz, Burns, & Williams, 1985; Zador, 1991). Persons at risk include young drivers who are inexperienced and tend to overestimate their driving skills. Members of this group are prone to risk-taking behaviors, including unsafe maneuvers and speeding, as well as much drinking on a single occasion. Worldwide, men are more involved in alcohol-related crashes. People with convictions for driving while under the influence are themselves frequent repeat offenders and are also more likely to be involved in fatal crashes (Beerman, Smith, & Hall, 1988; Perrine, 1990).

Note these other findings about blood-alcohol content (BAC): A 170-pound male would need to consume more than four drinks in an hour on an empty stomach to reach a BAC reading of 0.08 percent, the level at which a person is legally drunk. A 137-pound female would need three drinks in one hour on an empty stomach to reach that level. Most industrialized countries have set their legal BAC level at .08 percent or lower, but Australia, Finland, the Netherlands, and Norway have set it at .05, and Sweden has a legal BAC limit of .02. In other words, the Swedish authorities consider a blood-alcohol level at one-fourth of the U.S. drunk-driving limit to be dangerous (National Highway Traffic Safety Administration, 2000b). Reducing the legal driving BAC in a number of European countries resulted in fewer driving fatalities (Albalate, 2008). The European examples cited here are not isolated extremes—the U.S. level is in fact unusually lax when viewed in cross-national perspective.

In 1996, when five states in the United States reduced their BAC levels to 0.08 percent, a 16 percent reduction in alcohol-related fatal crashes resulted (Hingson, Heeren, & Winter, 1996). California experienced a 12 percent reduction in alcohol-related traffic deaths after it lowered its legal BAC limit to 0.08 percent. There was also an increase in arrests for driving under the influence (National Highway Traffic Safety Administration, 1994). Drunk-driving laws, which specify the length of time a license is administratively suspended following a DWI conviction, as well as interventions such as the use of alcohol interlock systems and other policies, vary from state to state. The Insurance Institute for Highway Safety has published a comprehensive listing of legal consequences for drunk driving.

According to the Centers for Disease Control and Prevention, effective means of reducing drunk driving accidents include the certainty of penalties, license revocation, graphic public service announcements and other media campaigns by Mothers Against Drunk Driving, sobriety checkpoints, alcohol-ignition-interlock programs, brief interventions and brief treatments of drunk drivers, responsible beverage service, and school-based programs about not being in a vehicle with an intoxicated driver (Transportation Research Board, 2003).

Evidence is inconclusive on the efficacy of designated-driver programs; a number of potential problems exist, including the possibility that the designated driver may also have been drinking (Ditter et al., 2005).

Politics of Drunk Driving

For 30 years, Mothers Against Drunk Driving (MADD) has been a major force in reducing vehicular fatalities due to drunk driving. Critics claim that the organization has lost the focus on drunk driving and instead is trying to reduce drinking in general. Some of the criticism has come from trade groups such as the American Beverage Institute (ABI), which claims that MADD and other so-called neo-prohibitionists are threatening the "on-premise dining experience, which often includes the responsible consumption of adult beverages." The following URLs provide examples of alcohol trade-group opposition to MADD initiatives: http://www.abi online.org and http://activistcash.com/organization_overview.cfm/o/17-mothers-against-drunk-driving.

The ABI opposes the .08 blood-alcohol limit for driving, increased sales tax on alcoholic beverages, and proposals for locking devices that prevent legally intoxicated drivers from starting their ignition. The ABI's Facebook page has a preponderance of postings opposing alcohol checkpoints for drivers.

According to a *New York Times* article in June 2010, although ABI is technically a nonprofit group, 82 percent of funds raised by the organization go to Berman and Co., a lobbyist group headed by Richard B. Berman (Strom, 2010).

Alcohol and Violence

The study of the interplay of alcohol and violence covers a broad spectrum of activities ranging from intimate partner violence and child abuse to brawls at bars and violence at sporting events. Interestingly, the latter factor is considered a major social problem in Europe but is relatively rare in America, where there is no equivalent of soccer hooligans (gangs or aggregates of individuals who travel to events with the intent of causing disturbances).

The availability of alcohol is related to violent assaults: The number of bars and liquor stores per capita is correlated to violent assault (Scribner, MacKinnon, & Dwyer, 1995), where industry is phased out and bars near factories close, murder rates drop, and alcohol sales at sporting events contribute to stadium violence.

In 1997, 40 percent of convicted rape and sexual-assault offenders said that they were drinking at the time of their crime (Greenfield &

Hennenberg, 1999). In 2002 more than 70,000 students ages 18–24 were victims of alcohol-related sexual assault in the United States (Hingson, Heeren, Zakocs, Kopstein, & Wechsler, 2002). In a study of police-citizen encounters, alcohol was present in 34 percent of these incidents. Violent encounters were 2.5 times more likely to involve alcohol than nonviolent encounters (McClelland & Teplin, 2001).

Many studies have correlated the relationship of alcohol and violence. A synthesis of studies commissioned for the International Center for Alcohol Policies, for example, concluded that both intoxication and psychological and cultural factors are involved in the link between alcohol and violence (Lennard, 2008). Other findings show that alcohol alone increases aggressive tendencies; alcohol coupled with the expectation of violence increases aggressive tendencies even more; with increased doses of alcohol, there is increased aggression; once aggression was initiated by intoxicated persons, it is less likely to be suppressed or limited; and intoxicated persons are more vulnerable to provocation and less able to think about the negatives consequences of their aggression (Yalisove, 2004).

Intimate-Partner Violence

Alcohol is strongly linked to intimate-partner violence. Women whose partners abuse alcohol are much more likely to be assaulted by their partners than other women (Kyriacou et al., 1999). Two-thirds of victims of domestic abuse have reported that alcohol was involved (Department of Justice, 2010). Factors that determine the strong link between alcohol and intimate partner violence include the disinhibitory effect of alcohol; depression of functions in the cerebral cortex that govern rational problem solving and judgment; belief in the disinhibitory effect that creates a set, a rationale, and an expectation of violence; cultural beliefs in the appropriateness of male violence toward female partners and/or its demonstration of masculinity; heavy drinking that can create stressors in relationships because of economic hardships, infidelities, and so forth; and use of alcohol as a method of coping when violence occurs in a relationship (Finney, 2003).

Other co-occurring psychiatric disorders, other than substance abuse, make the risk of violence greater. Antisocial personality disorder in men is one of the most frequently associated conditions. Heavy drinkers may antagonize their partners due to failure to meet responsibilities and because of drunken behavior. Their personal hygiene may be spotty, and their romantic behavior and sexual advances will be crude. Partner disinterest may lead to paranoid imaginings and even violence. The alcoholic may imagine, as well, that his or her entire family is conspiring against him or her (Foran & O'Leary, 2008).

Sociocultural factors have a major influence on the connection between alcohol and violence. (See Part II, 4b.) Rates of alcohol consumption do *not* correlate to rates of violence in many nations. For example, Luxembourg has one of the highest rates of alcohol consumption but a low rate of violence. In a cross-cultural study of alcohol and violence, it has been found that cultural features contribute to a link between alcohol and violence. These include cultural support for aggression and aggressive solutions to interpersonal problems (as in the media and in folklore), militaristic and warlike culture, glorification of fighters and fighting, violent sports, the socialization of male children toward aggressiveness, an unusually high proportion of young males in the society, and beliefs that alcohol or specific beverages make one behave badly or cause domestic violence (Fox, 2008, pp. 15–16).

Alcohol in the Workplace

Alcohol use in the workplace, or at lunch breaks, affects safety, productivity, and efficiency. Workplace accidents are associated with drinking on the job or during lunch breaks, increasing health costs to employers, including disability and workers'-compensation claims. Heavy drinking after hours results in workers showing up with hangovers that impact safety, productivity, and efficiency, not to mention lateness and absenteeism. The alcohol-abusing worker shifts jobs much more often than the sober worker, often quitting just before termination takes place (Institute of Alcohol Studies, 2009).

Workplace cultures of drinking are associated with alcohol abuse on the job. These may involve supervisors who have risen from the ranks and who maintain their peer or quasi-peer status. They are unlikely to discourage workplace drinking and unlikely to refer employees to employee-assistance programs for alcohol abuse and dependency. Workplace drinking, largely but not exclusively a male activity, acts to proclaim, bond, and reaffirm social solidarity among peers.

Workplace alienation is another major factor in drinking on the job. Alienation is a result of boredom, stress and repetitiveness in job tasks, the worker's lack of autonomy and lack of control over industrial or other work processes and conditions, and estrangement from others. Although issues of worker alienation were traditionally associated with the early teachings of Karl Marx in the mid-19th century, the National Institute for Alcoholism and Alcohol Abuse cites alienation as a factor in workplace drinking problems (National Institute on Alcohol Abuse and Alcoholism, 1999a).

The phrase "employee-assistance programs" (EAPs) often euphemistically refers to alcohol- and drug-intervention programs. Ordinarily, they concentrate on alcohol and other drug problems, but broad-brush EAPs also concern themselves with mental health, family, and other problem areas. EAPs screen and assess individuals for substance-related problems and refer them for treatment to outside agencies. Although many people self-refer to EAPs, involuntary referrals from supervisors or from human resources departments also occur.

OTHER PROBLEMS

As we have documented above, alcohol is associated with huge costs to society and deaths to drivers, passengers, and people in other vehicles, and it contributes to a large proportion of violent personal encounters with partners and strangers and is a source of workplace problems. We will now briefly summarize some adverse consequences to intoxication that are not reported as often.

Accidents not involving motor vehicles occur at substantially high rates to individuals engaged in heavy drinking. These include falls and boating accidents (Howland & Hingson, 1987; Johnston & McGovern, 2004). Alcoholics are ten times more likely than the general population to suffer burns and, when burned, to suffer fatal burns. A significant portion of these injuries and deaths are due to falling asleep drunk while smoking (Howland & Hingson, 1987). Also, during the heat wave of 2010, dozens of Russians drowned each day; 1,200 deaths occurred in June alone. Vadim Seryogin of Russia's Emergencies Ministry was widely quoted in the media as stating, "The majority of those drowned were drunk" (ABC Online, 2010). They drank, usually vodka, before swimming, and many drank while in the water. Children also drowned, because their families, camp counselors, and other caretakers were drinking or drunk. These drowning-while-intoxicated figures are not matched in other nations that do not have a tradition of drinking and swimming.

Levels of drinking are highly correlated to delinquent behaviors by youth, including property damage, fights in school, group-against-group fights, and stealing (National Survey on Drug Use and Health, 2005). So-called secondhand drinking—the term is derived from an analogy to secondhand smoke—includes humiliation and embarrassment, having an argument, being kept up at night, being insulted or harassed, or being pushed or hit (Wechsler & Kuo, 2000); alcohol abuse is also implicated in sex crimes, unwanted sexual encounters, suicide, and child abuse, which are discussed later in this volume.

CHAPTER 7

Alcohol and Medical Problems

Beverage alcohol is the drug most deleterious to health, except for cigarettes, far outweighing the damage done by heroin, cocaine, or other illicit drugs. It is also remarkable in the health consequences to so many diverse biochemical and organ systems. It has been said that "to know alcohol is to know medicine" (anonymous). It is paradoxical that alcohol-related disease is treated, yet the alcohol misuse itself is largely not. A physician recovering from alcoholism called this the ash can syndrome: A man found passed out in an alley among the ash cans (no longer prevalent in post-coal America) is treated for infections, gastritis, malnutrition, blood disorders, and hepatitis, but not for the alcoholism that undergirded these problems.

THE ALIMENTARY CANAL

The esophagus, or gullet, a sensitive organ covered by a mucous membrane, is the muscular tube that conveys solids and liquids from the back of the throat to the stomach. The immediate effect of alcohol ingestion is to irritate the mucosa. The warm feeling created by drinking a strong alcoholic beverage is, in fact, irritation. Continued irritation, known as esophagitis, can be a minor cause of esophageal bleeding. Alcoholism is also associated with elevated rates of esophageal cancer due to prolonged esophagitis.

Alcohol also irritates the stomach, a condition known as gastritis. Furthermore, alcohol consumption results in production of more gastric (stomach) acid, which can compound gastritis and contribute to peptic ulcers and potential bleeding. (Ulcers are also caused by gastric bacteria.) Alcoholism is also associated with elevated rates of stomach cancer due to prolonged gastritis.

The pyloric valve stops or allows food and fluids to leave the stomach for the small intestine. At high concentrations, alcohol paralyzes the pyloric valve. The backup of stomach contents, together with gastritis, causes nausea and vomiting, and contributes to further esophagitis and some esophageal bleeding.

Gastric hyperacidity can also irritate the duodenum, the first segment of the small intestine, and can contribute to the formation of a peptic ulcer and bleeding. Irritation of the large, or lower, intestine leads to diarrhea. Alcoholic diarrhea and vomiting lead to dehydration and potassium depletion.

THE PANCREAS

The pancreas is a small organ located near the bottom of the stomach. Its two functions are to produce digestive juices containing enzymes that digest starch, break down fats, and process protein and to secrete the hormones insulin, which brings blood sugar levels down, and glucagons, which raises blood sugar levels.

Pancreatitis, or inflammation of the pancreas, can occur for several reasons, including the production of gallstones (cholelithiasis) and alcohol abuse. About one-third of pancreatitis cases are due to alcohol abuse and alcoholism. Nausea, vomiting, fever, and abdominal pain are typical manifestations of acute pancreatitis. Although pancreatitis can often be treated and relieved, permanent damage to the pancreas can be fatal; even recovering alcoholics die of pancreatitis they contracted while they were actively addicted.

Chronic pancreatitis causes malabsorption of nutrients, weight loss, and malnourishment because the digestive enzymes are not available. The other condition associated with alcoholic pancreatitis is alcoholic diabetes. Diabetes is a disease of abnormally high blood sugar, in this case related to the inability of the pancreas to provide insulin.

THE LIVER

A majority of deaths resulting from chronic alcohol abuse have to do with alcoholic liver disease. The liver is an organ located in the upper right-hand portion of the abdominal cavity, beneath the diaphragm, on top of the stomach. Hundreds of important physiological functions are performed by the liver, including

- production of bile that breaks down fats in the small intestine.
- production of cholesterol and special proteins to help carry fats through the body.

- conversion of glucose into glycogen that can later be converted back to glucose for energy.
- the processing of hemoglobin for iron in the body.
- iron storage.
- conversion of poisonous ammonia to harmless urea, which is excreted in urine, and detoxifying other toxins, including psychoactive drugs.
- regulating blood clotting.
- helping the body resist infections by producing immune factors and removing bacteria from the blood.

Forms of Alcoholic Liver Disease

Alcoholic hepatitis, or liver inflammation due to heavy drinking, is but one of the several forms of hepatitis that include the viral forms hepatitis A, B, C, and D. An alcoholic may have hepatitis B or C in addition to bouts of alcoholic hepatitis because B and C are spread through sexual contact or through infected needles. They, like alcoholic hepatitis, cause liver damage. (Hepatitis C is the most serious of the viral varieties.) Symptoms of alcoholic hepatitis include jaundice (a yellowish tinge of the skin and in the whites of the eyes), fatigue, fever, nausea and loss of appetite, vomiting, and abdominal pain. About one-third of heavy drinkers have bouts of hepatitis that are usually treatable. The drinker must abstain, however.

Fatty liver, or build-up of fat in the liver cells, can cause discomfort in the upper stomach and enlargement of the liver.

Alcoholic cirrhosis of the liver is an irreversible scarring of the liver resulting from years of heavy drinking, contraction of chronic hepatitis B or C, or exposure to toxic chemicals. Depending on the population, 10–20 percent of long-term heavy drinkers develop some degree of cirrhosis. Healthy liver cells (hepatocytes) are gradually replaced by scar tissue as cells die from chronic inflammation. High concentrations of ethanol also contribute to iron deposits in the liver, which adds another toxicity factor. Often, this condition is only diagnosed postmortem, by biopsy (Johns Hopkins, 2011).

There are several serious and life-threatening consequences of cirrhosis: The liver fails to clear toxins such as ammonia from the blood, which then travel to the brain, causing cognitive disturbances, confusion, coma, and death. (This is known as hepatic encephalopathy, a common cause of death from alcoholism.) Also, bruising and bleeding occurs as the liver fails to produce proteins necessary for blood clotting; the spleen becomes enlarged; fewer platelets are found in the blood (low platelet count often leads physicians to look for cirrhosis); the immune system is compromised and bacteria are not cleared from blood, leading to infections that are difficult to heal. In addition, kidney failure (hepatrenal syndrome) and lung failure (hepatopulmonary syndrome) occur; more cases of liver cancer occur among alcohol abusers than in the nonalcoholic population; and blood backs up in the large vein leading to the liver and in the tributaries of that vein, a condition known as portal-vein hypertension.

Portal-vein hypertension itself has various consequences, including ascites, or the filling of the abdominal cavity with fluid (University of Washington, 2011); swelling (varicose) veins in the esophagus, which that can burst under pressure, a life threatening event (see figure 7.1); swollen (varicose) veins in the stomach; bleeding hemorrhoids; distorted and engorged veins spreading out from the center of the stomach; and spiderlike veins radiating from elevated red spots (spider angioma) (Merck 2011).

Once cirrhosis and its complications develop, the five-year survival rate is about 50 percent. Abstention from alcohol raises that rate. Liver transplantation is a successful treatment for cirrhosis. Two of the more prominent persons to receive a liver transplant for alcoholic cirrhosis are Mickey Mantle, Hall of Fame baseball player for the New York Yankees, and

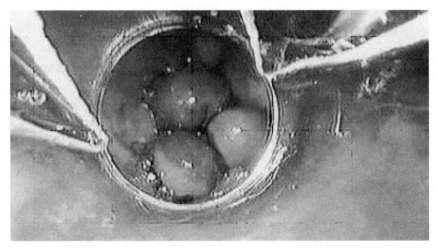

Figure 7.1 View of varices in the esophagus, a consequence of liver disease, using endoscopy. These dilated veins are being banded to prevent gastrointestinal bleeding.

Source: Marsano et al. (2003).

singer/guitarist David Crosby of The Byrds and Crosby, Stills and Nash; these cases created controversies over the fairness of the liver-allocation system and whether they were appropriate candidates. Most transplant programs require six months of abstinence prior to performing the surgery.

NERVOUS SYSTEM
Acute Effects of Alcohol on the Brain

The major structures of the brain are all affected by alcohol in roughly the following order (see also figure 7.2):

- The cerebral cortex, involved in judgment, thinking, perception, and cognition, is suppressed by relatively low doses of alcohol, resulting in disinhibited behavior, poor judgment, and poor choices. Ridiculous behavior at office parties, misperception and evaluation of sexual signals, and other complications in interpersonal and social situations are typical outcomes.

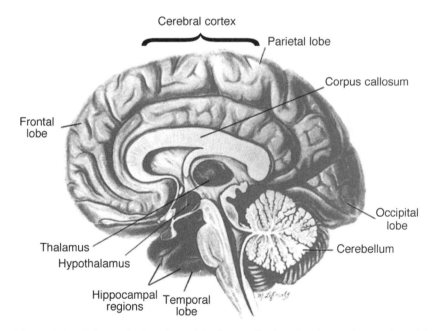

Figure 7.2 Schematic drawing of the human brain, showing regions vulnerable to alcoholism-related abnormalities.

Source: National Institute on Alcohol and Alcoholism, U.S. National Institutes of Health.

- The cerebellum, involved in gross motor behavior, is suppressed at higher doses, resulting in slurred speech and staggering gait and deficiencies in driving skills.
- The medulla and other parts of the brain stem are suppressed at very high doses, resulting in unconsciousness, respiratory depression, and death (Zealberg & Brady, 1999).

Alcohol and Sleep

Another acute effect of alcohol relates to sleep. Alcohol promotes sleepiness and sleep but disrupts the sleep cycle. In sleep, the brain is actually quite active, and sleep has important psychological and physiological functions. One of the functions alcohol suppresses is REM, or dream, sleep (named after the rapid eye movements and the dreams that occur during this state). Being passed out from alcohol has more in common with a person hit over the head or knocked out in a prizefight than the complex rhythms of normal, restorative sleep. Episodes of waking during the night are also increased. A person does not wake up refreshed and clear from alcoholic sleep.

BLACKOUTS

The so-called alcohol blackout is a period of time in which a person who has become intoxicated cannot remember events. This is an alcohol-induced amnesia caused by the brain's inability to encode memories due to high concentrations of alcohol in the blood. It can be total, exemplified in the phenomenon informally known as the lost weekend, or partial. A person who drinks a lot in a short period of time and on an empty stomach is more likely to experience a blackout. Although many people consider the blackout a warning sign of developing alcoholism, this is not necessarily the case. In a study of college students who were asked, "Have you ever awoken after a night of drinking not able to remember things that you did or places that you went?" 51 percent of student drinkers reported having experienced such a blackout, and 40 percent reported blacking out in the current year. Most alarmingly, of those who had been drinking during the two weeks prior to the survey, almost 10 percent had blacked out. Many reported finding out that they had participated in behavior such as vandalism and unprotected sex (White, 2003; White, Jamieson-Drake, & Swartzwelder, 2002). In blackouts, some drinkers act normally, others engage in intoxicated behaviors such as the students in the White studies, and still others engage in bizarre behaviors such as taking a bus to another city, where they emerge from their blackout state.

ALCOHOLIC BRAIN SYNDROMES

Wernicke's encephalopathy is a condition caused by the failure of the alcohol abuser to take in and absorb Vitamin B_1, or niacin, which impairs and destroys neurons on the brain. It is marked by eye-movement disorders, double vision, movement disorders such as ataxia, or staggering, sluggishness, inattentiveness, confusion, and memory loss.

Korsakoff's psychosis, now thought to be part of an overall Wernicke-Korsakoff syndrome, has notable symptom confabulation—making up stories and accounts of things that did not happen—which is important to distinguish from confabulation found in senile dementia. Treatment with niacin can clear up much of the eye and movement problems but not the inability to store memories. Alcohol-induced persisting amnestic disorder or wet brain are other terms for Wernicke-Korsakoff syndrome.

Atrophy of the cerebral cortex, especially the prefrontal cortex, which is the brain's executive center, compromises planning and regulating behavior, inhibition of inappropriate behavior, and, in general, negatively affects skills such as goal-directed behavior, problem solving, and judgment. Thus, some antisocial behaviors, as well as overall deterioration in functioning and even inability to realize the gravity of one's situation, can be chalked up to this real brain damage (Oscar-Berman & Marinkovic, 2003).

Cerebellar degeneration (of the cerebellum) causes tremors and severe coordination limitations of the lower extremities. This condition and Wernicke's syndrome contribute to a rickety, wide-based so-called sailor's gait in alcoholics even when they are not drinking.

Alcoholic peripheral neuropathy is a disorder of decreased nerve function due to the damage of alcohol abuse. Because alcoholics drink empty calories, because the liver processes alcohol preferably over other nutrients, and because of malabsorption of nutrients in the alcoholic's body, vitamin deficiencies negatively affect nerve cells in muscles. Nerves that control movement and sensation are affected *and* symptoms of this syndrome include numbness in the arms and legs, abnormal sensations and the feeling that one is being stuck by pins and needles, painful sensations in the arms and legs, muscle weakness, muscle cramps or muscle aches, male impotence, and incontinence (leaking urine).

One of the most common alcoholic brain-related deaths, mentioned in the section on the liver, is hepatic, or portosystemic, encephalopathy, in which liver failure causes toxins to build up in the brain. Finally, because the nerve cells are not firing properly, atrophy of the musculature of the arms and legs often occurs.

In the advanced alcoholic, there is the characteristic look of the swollen abdomen from ascites, described above, coupled with skinny arms and legs, and the odd, rolling sailors gait.

THE BLOOD AND HEART

Many blood functions are affected by alcoholism: red blood cells, responsible for carrying oxygen, are not produced normally, leading to anemia, and white blood cells, responsible for fighting infection, are not produced normally, leading to infections that develop frequently and are slow to heal. The risk of infections in patients undergoing cardiac surgery is raised fourfold among long-term alcoholics. Platelets, responsible for blood clotting, are not produced normally, leading to bleeding disorders (Fleming, Milic, & Harris, 2006; Sander, 2005). A heavy drinker is, of course, at risk for falling and striking his or her head, or suffering a head impact in an auto accident. Therefore, heavy drinkers are at risk for brain bleeding and subdural hematomas, or blood clots under the skull. The symptoms associated with this condition, drifting in and out of consciousness, might be hard to distinguish from those of ordinary severe intoxication.

Cardiovascular System

Prolonged, heavy alcohol intake can damage cells of the heart muscle, leading to a weakened, enlarged heart, a form of heart failure known as alcoholic cardiomyopathy. (See figure 7.3.) Alcohol abuse accounts for only a small percentage of cases of heart failure (Rubin & Doria, 1990). It is identical in symptoms to heart failure due to viral infection, high blood pressure, and so on and is the basis for shortness of breath, poor oxygenation of the body, and potentially fatal arrhythmias, or abnormal heart rhythms.

Moderate drinking (i.e., two drinks per day) lowers the risk of coronary artery disease. However, hypertension (high blood pressure) is found one and one half to two times more in men who drink more than five drinks per day (Klatsky, 1996). Red wine, in particular, has antioxidants that are thought to protect the linings of the blood vessels from inflammation. Binge drinking may also precipitate arrhythmias such as atrial fibrillation in otherwise healthy individuals. This condition, associated with holiday drinking, is known colloquially as holiday heart.

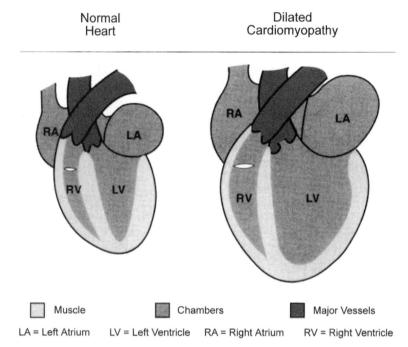

Figure 7.3   A heart in dilated cardiomyopathy compared with a normal heart at end systole (end of contraction).

Source: National Institute on Alcohol and Alcoholism, U.S. National Institutes of Health.

WITHDRAWAL SYNDROMES

Uncomplicated Acute Alcohol Withdrawal, or Alcohol-Abstinence Syndrome

Alcohol is a depressant, and the central-nervous-system (CNS) functions of the person who drinks heavily and continuously are chronically depressed. When the alcoholic abstains for whatever reason, the CNS bounces back like a spring in a mattress when you get out of bed. This rebound hyperactivity causes symptoms that include anxiety, the shakes (tremor in the hands), irritability, tachyocardia (rapid heartbeat), loss of appetite, insomnia, and nightmares when sleep does occur.

Withdrawal syndromes can happen upon awakening and/or when the blood-alcohol level is low. With prolonged drinking and development of metabolic tolerance, the drinker can go into withdrawal even with a moderate amount of alcohol in the blood. One of the vicious cycles in the development of alcoholism occurs this way when the alcohol abuser is prompted to have a morning drink to ward off the shakes. Hangover cures that include a drink—the source of the expression "the hair of the dog that bit me"—are a trap for the unwary. Uncomplicated alcohol withdrawal should run its course in three days, although sleep disturbances can continue for some time. A problem associated with abstinence is that other medical conditions that have been masked will now make their presence known.

Withdrawal with Complications, or Major Withdrawal

A complication that occurs in about one-fifth of people undergoing withdrawal, alcoholic hallucinosis, or auditory and visual hallucinations and severe nightmares, may come on after a day into withdrawal and can be a short-term or chronic condition.

Withdrawal seizures, known colloquially as rum fits, which resemble standard grand mal epileptic seizures and last about a minute, can come on within 12–48 hours into withdrawal for a minority of people. Emergency physicians need to rule out many other conditions that could precipitate seizures among drinkers, such as subdural hematomas, conditions unrelated to drinking, or conditions that are aggravated by drinking, such as the lower seizure threshold for epileptics in the morning.

Delirium Tremens (DTs)

Delirium tremens, colloquially known as having the DTs, is the most severe complication of withdrawal. It is a life-threatening condition if untreated that includes fever, disorientations, seizures, hallucinations, confusion and paranoia, and elevated blood pressure. In literature, it is sometimes called the horrors. Mark Twain depicted DTs in *Huckleberry Finn:* Huck's father, an alcoholic, passes out drunk but awakes with full-fledged DTs. The stereotyped victim of DTs sees pink elephants; Walt Disney's *Fantasia* depicts Mickey Mouse having these hallucinations after a drinking bout (Fleming et al., 2006).

(Note: It is not within the scope of this volume to describe the vast number of rare medical conditions associated with alcoholism.)

ALCOHOL-USE DISORDERS AND CO-OCCURRING PSYCHIATRIC DISORDERS

It is a historical curiosity that the psychiatry and alcoholism treatment were separate streams of effort for many decades, involving separate treatment personnel and facilities, beliefs, and techniques. Training for mental health professionals and for addictions counselors usually gave little thought to the other wing of the helping professions. Contributing to this divide was the perception by many medical personnel that alcoholics were uncooperative and difficult to treat and could or would not pay. Moreover, alcoholism treatment emerged from self-help movements, and alcoholics felt that medicine had failed them, if not mistreated them, before they entered into recovery through self-help groups. That history is detailed later in this volume.

For alcoholics who suffered from another behavioral or mental health issue as well, the problems were worse; they belonged to two stigmatized social categories, they were shuttled back and forth between psychiatric and addictions treatment, and they were often misdiagnosed, or were discharged from treatment as soon as they were stabilized for the moment, without their deep-set issues being addressed. Treatment professionals, dedicated as they might be, felt frustrated at the chronic, recurring, cyclic nature of their problems, the poor prognosis, and the noncompliance and behavioral disorganization of a person with mental illness added on to alcoholism (Myers & Salt, 2007).

Starting in the 1990s, these treatment efforts began to merge into an integrated, comprehensive system of care. It is now understood that dual diagnoses (having a psychiatric disorder on top of a substance-use disorder) are the norm, not the exception. Alcohol abusers and alcoholics experience many psychiatric problems, not all of which are within the scope of this volume.

Schizophrenia is a neurodevelopmental, biologically based brain disorder marked by distorted information processing, including delusions and hallucinations, as well as bizarre behavior and severe apathy.

According to noted schizophrenia researcher Nancy Andreasen (1999), schizophrenia results from some combination of inherited neurobiological vulnerability and a number of environmental risk factors that may affect the fetus, often in the second trimester. Schizophrenia has symptoms that include hallucinations (usually auditory, such as hearing voices), delusions such as that a television announcer is talking directly to the hallucinator, or paranoid delusions such as that the person is the target of a vast conspiracy or that he or she is of divine or royal origin. The schizophrenic often has bizarre and/or disorganized speech and behavior and appears to have a flat emotional presentation and extreme apathy. The onset of schizophrenia is often in the late teens and early adulthood, which is also the time that individuals are at high risk for alcohol and other drug abuse. Schizophrenics may find that drinking helps them numb the terrors and chaos that prevail in their inner psychic experience. Schizophrenia is not caused in any way by alcohol or other drugs, but heavy drinking certainly contributes to the instability of a person having great difficulty in living a normal life.

Mood Disorders

Mood disorders include depression and bipolar disorder, or manic depression. Depression has many causes, including genetic predisposition, trauma, unresolved grief, external stressors, and helpless, hopeless patterns of thinking and behavior. Many depressed people drink to blot out the bad feelings they experience, but alcohol is a depressant drug that may allow them to be momentarily numb but not happy. Medications for the treatment of depression cannot have their proper effect in the presence of high blood-alcohol levels, and, as noted previously, the medical, social, and psychological consequences of alcohol abuse inflict considerable pain, a vicious cycle in the life of a depressed alcohol abuser. Alcohol, as also previously noted, harms the quality of sleep, contributing to depression. Alcohol puts the drinker at risk for depression as much as the reverse (Fergusson, Boden, & Horwood, 2009).

Bipolar disorder involving severe and extreme mood swings. The bipolar individual often drinks to come down from a manic state, as well as to blot out depressive symptoms when on the other leg of the mood swing. About one-half of people with bipolar disorder have an alcohol-use disorder (Sonne & Brady, 2001).

Posttraumatic stress disorder (PTSD) may involve hypervigilance, insomnia, reexperiencing of the traumatic event or events, or flashbacks, or emotional numbness. People who have experienced abuse or been victims of a crime or a catastrophe, or people who have lived through war and/ or genocide, can experience PTSD. Many alcoholism inpatient units of the Veterans Administration hospital system are populated with veterans with both alcohol and PTSD disorders (Substance Abuse Mental Health Services Administration, n.d.).

Attention-deficit hyperactivity disorder (ADHD) involves some combination of physical and mental hyperactivity and the inability to focus, attend, and organize. People with ADHD may be very intelligent, but may have severe academic problems such as the inability to finish written work. People with the symptoms of ADHD experience failure, rejection, and low self-esteem. They will drink to calm down, to sleep, and to numb their bad feelings. They will also tend to gravitate to others who are substance abusers (Smith, Molina, & Pelham, 2002).

Personality Disorders

A wide variety of personality disorders exist, but the ones most associated with alcohol abuse are the antisocial personality disorder and the borderline personality disorder. The person with antisocial personality disorder feels few inhibitions about engaging in socially deviant behavior and violence, and feels no remorse upon completion. This behavior dovetails or worsens the connections between alcohol and violence documented earlier in this section. The person with borderline personality disorder has great swings in mood and attitude, engages in self-destructive acts, has very unstable relationships, and is prone to overreact to small real or imagined slights. Those with this condition may flip from idealizing a person one day to devaluing them the next day, and may have an emotional amnesia about prior attitudes. This is a profile not unlike the alcoholic, who has mood swings, blackouts, and impulsive and self-destructive behaviors, so it is hard to sort out what symptoms stems from chemical abuse or from personality organization or are behaviors influenced by both (Myers, 2008).

Alcohol and Suicide

Suicide, as well as suicidal gestures, are related to a wide range of social and cultural factors, and studies done on alcohol and suicide in one nation may not pertain to other nations. In a study of 13 European nations, suicide was positively correlated to per capita alcohol use in 10 of the countries. In individuals with major depression or personality disorders (especially borderline personality disorder), impulsivity, and aggressive tendencies, the correlations with suicidality rise significantly. Various studies have shown from one-third to two-thirds of completed suicides were legally intoxicated, and perhaps one-fifth of all alcoholically dependent individuals commit suicide. Being male and over the age of 50 also increases the rates of suicide while intoxicated (Preuss, Koller, Barnow, Eikmeier, & Soyka, 2006; Sher, 2005). Alcohol-related disappointments such as divorce or loss of a job, and resultant isolation, are also associated factors, especially in the older male with an alcohol-use disorder (Kendall, 1983).

CONCLUSION

Overall, the relationship between alcohol use disorders and other behavioral and psychiatric disorders is quite complex:

- Alcoholism may aid in the reemergence of psychiatric disorders that had been stabilized.
- Alcoholism may worsen existing psychiatric disorders.
- Alcoholism may mimic some symptoms of psychiatric disorders.
- Paradoxically, alcoholism may help to mask, dampen, or disguise psychiatric disorders. It may seem to offer some sense of control,

while the underlying problem is not addressed or worsened. After detoxification, a person may feel the full force of his or her mental illness, prompting the desire to start drinking again.

- Alcohol-withdrawal syndromes may resemble psychiatric disorders.
- Psychiatric disorders increase the risk of alcoholism.
- Side effects of psychiatric medications may resemble those caused by psychiatric symptoms or substance abuse.
- The relative importance of alcoholism or other co-occurring disorders may wax or wane (Myers & Salt, 2007).

CHAPTER 8

Alcohol and Sexuality

Alcohol is a paradoxical substance when it comes to sex. It generates a lot of sexual behavior, but much of it is unwanted or regretted, and much of it is impaired. Shakespeare said this well a full 400 years ago, as did a 20th-century blues singer:

> [Alcohol] provokes and unprovokes; it provokes the desire, but it takes away the performance.
>
> —William Shakespeare, *Macbeth* II, 3

> Me and my woman on a drinking spree, I can't find her and she can't find me.
>
> —Toombs (1953)

SEXUAL PHARMACOLOGY

At moderate doses, both males and females report experiencing heightened sexual arousal (Crenshaw & Goldberg, 1996; Goldman & Roehrich, 1991). This experience can be due to the disinhibiting effect of alcohol, the suppression of anxiety about socializing and about sexuality, and the suppression of guilt.

In addition, alcohol impacts how we process information. Impairment of attention to information about what is appropriate or safe behavior, and to possible consequences such as pregnancies or sexually transmitted disease, occur. There is an appraisal and a definition of the alcohol-using situation as giving one permission for rule breaking, where one can neglect to attend to important information about what is appropriate and safe—a so-called time out.

Risky sexual behaviors and sexual behaviors that in retrospect would seem undesirable are more likely to occur at elevated blood-alcohol levels. This is applicable for people normally fearful about sexual risk taking who acquire what is known as liquid courage (Stoner, George, Norris, & Peters, 2007).

When male experimental subjects are given nonalcoholic drinks but are told the drinks *are* alcoholic, they report increased sexual arousal. This reminds us of the famous quote, "What we believe to be true is true in its social consequences." This effect does not occur in females, however, at least not in an experimental setting (Goldman & Roehrich, 1991). What psychologists call alcohol expectancies is similar to what sociologists and anthropologists call drunken comportment, discussed in later section on alcohol and culture.

Males and females who have had high doses of alcohol experience a reduction in sexual arousal and performance, and in this case, erections for males and orgasms for both males and females are less likely.

Reproductive hormone production is impaired by chronic heavy drinking, resulting in sexual dysfunction and infertility. Alcohol is toxic to the testes, which produce the male hormone testosterone. Male alcoholics often have erectile disorders, and some display feminization characteristics such as breast enlargement. Alcohol is also toxic to the ovaries. Reproductive disorders, cessation of menstruation, menstrual irregularity, failure to ovulate, and spontaneous abortion may occur in women who drink heavily, even among those who do not meet the criteria for diagnosis as alcohol abusers or alcoholics (National Institute on Alcohol Abuse and Alcoholism, 1994).

Sexual behavior is also affected due to the difficulty in finding or successfully maintaining sexual and/or romantic partners when alcoholism causes deterioration.

ALCOHOL AND UNWANTED SEXUAL ENCOUNTERS

Approximately one-fourth of American women have experienced sexual assault. In about half of these cases, alcohol was consumed by the perpetrator, the victim, or both. These figures are tentative, because most sexual assault goes unreported for a variety of reasons. Among them, many women blame themselves for having been drunk when victimized and may not even categorize the event as rape or assault.

Abbey and colleagues (2001) have identified several stages of interaction in which cues are misread, leading to the likelihood of sexual assault. Alcohol contributes to misreading of women's behavior, so that men, due to diminished cognitive function, may perceive women as encouraging sex. Women, also experiencing worsened cognitive functioning, don't perceive the danger in the situation, and don't realize they have not made it clear to a man that they are not interested. Women who have been drinking tend to be blamed for encouraging sexual assault more than women who have not been drinking. This phenomenon is more pronounced in interracial rather than intraracial situations (George & Martinez, 2002).

Male perpetrators of sexual assault are more hostile toward women and lower in empathy than other men, more likely than others to hold to outdated stereotypes about gender roles, more likely to endorse statements that justify rape such as that women enjoy forced sex, and more often to view relationships between the sexes as adversarial (Seto & Barabee, 1997). Gender attitudes, roles, and beliefs vary tremendously across cultural boundaries, and thus culture figures into any equation concerning sexual assault.

ALCOHOL AND SEXUALLY TRANSMITTED DISEASES

Level of alcohol use is directly correlated to the incidence and prevalence of sexually transmitted disease. (See figure 8.1.) Out of all young adults, 1.4 percent have STDs, but 2.5 percent of heavy drinkers have STDs. Research that shows that alcohol abuse increases the risk of and spread of HIV/AIDS (National Institute on Alcohol Abuse and Alcoholism, 2002).

MISPERCEPTION OF SOCIAL SIGNALS, AND BEER GOGGLES

Experimental research has validated the common belief that alcohol influence people to find members of the opposite sex more attractive, leading to the possibility of risky sex or sex they will regret (Jones, Jones, Thomas, & Piper, 2003). In one experimental study by Parker and colleagues (2008), subjects rated the faces people of the opposite or same sex as more attractive when intoxicated, and men who rated women as more attractive while intoxicated maintained that rating when questioned 24 hours later. The perception of attractiveness seemed to have been encoded in their brains, and they recalled the females as attractive even when sober the following day. This recalled attractiveness did not occur with female subjects, however.

In separate research, Abbey and colleagues (2000) found that alcohol influenced the perception of sexual availability. When a couple drank together, they rated themselves and their partner as more sexual and

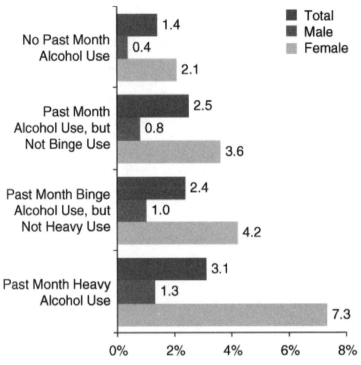

Figure 8.1   Relationship of drinking to rates of sexually transmitted disease.

Source: Substance Abuse and Mental Health Services Administration (2007).

disinhibited. Males tended to ignore signals from women that indicated they were not interested in sex. Women who are drinking are perceived as less attractive. Interestingly, alcohol does not affect men's ability to judge the age of a woman, so beer goggles cannot be blamed for men engaging in sex with minors (Egan & Cordan, 2009).

CHAPTER 9

Alcohol and the Family

According to one estimate (Grant et al., 2006), one-half of all families in the nation have or have had a member with an alcohol-use disorder. In many of these families, the disorder becomes the central issue around which the family must adjust to or organize itself. Inadequate or abusive parenting, maladaptive roles for children and spouses, and unhealthy and destructive communication patterns often ensue. Much popular literature in the late 20th century focused on such concepts as codependence and adult children of alcoholics.

OVERVIEW OF EFFECTS OF ALCOHOL ON THE FAMILY

The scope of alcohol abuse as a problem for families is immense. Alcoholism can take a devastating toll on the family. For example, parental alcohol abuse may increase the chance that a child will experience physical and/or sexual abuse either by a family member or a stranger (Widom & Hiller-Sturmhofel, 2001). Not only is alcohol an emotional and behavioral disinhibitor, but, when intoxicated, an individual misinterprets social cues, misperceives threats, and does not recognize the consequences of violence. A person who is violent when intoxicated may minimize his or her own responsibility for the consequence of violence (Miller, Maguin, & Down, 1997). Alcoholic blackouts may also occur during physical and sexual abuse, and an intoxicated parent may hit a baby that is colicky or cries inconsolably. In addition, abused children are themselves at risk for adult alcohol-use disorders (Widom & Hiller-Sturmhofel, 2001; Widom, White, Czaja, & Marmorstein, 2007).

Parenting by alcohol abusers can be chaotic, inconsistent, and unpredictable. The alcohol-abusing parent is less likely to provide appropriate feeding and bedtime routines infants need, to cope with infants' nighttime awakenings, and to provide correct nutrition. As children of alcoholics enter school, there is less likelihood that they will receive adequate help with or monitoring of homework or that parents will attend parent-teacher conferences. As a teenager, in fact, the child of an alcoholic will wish to shield outsiders from knowledge of familial alcoholism. Various patterns of alcoholic parental behavior emerge; to cite but one, there is the parent who engages in weekend binge drinking, feels guilty and hung over on Monday, and engages in a semblance of normal functioning midweek.

Communication patterns in the alcoholic family are disrupted; there is a heightened possibility of verbally aggressive and hostile interactions and/ or emotional withdrawal. Black (2002) identified communication roles in the alcoholic family as "Don't talk, don't trust, don't feel." Certainly, a loving family environment is made less likely. Members often feel shameful, incompetent, helpless and hopeless, and traumatized.

Alcoholism is the elephant in the room. Alcoholism itself and the negative consequences it engenders are family secrets. The family tends to circle the wagons, withdrawing from interaction with outsiders. There is a discrepancy in the face it offers the world (the front stage) and the inner life of the family (the backstage). And although they may not be aware of it, family members may engage in behavior that actually encourages the alcohol abuse of its drinking member. This is known in the recovery community as enabling. Examples include

- making excuses for drinkers such as calling in to work sick for them or using illness as a reason for absence from an occasion such as a wedding or a dinner party
- bailing them out when they are arrested for drunk and disorderly behavior
- taking them in from the street, where they have passed out, and putting them to bed
- giving them money the nondrinker knows will be spent on liquor
- denying or minimizing the problem to others in the family and to health care providers and other helping professionals

Enabling behaviors have the effect of preventing alcohol abusers from facing the reality and consequences of their alcohol use, buffering them from the shocks that would befall them. This is a case in which helping actually hurts. Family members fear to stop enabling and will keep the status quo at all costs. In this way, they participate in the addiction themselves, a state known in the recovery community as codependency. Family life tends to revolve around the alcoholism itself, an unhealthy situation in which lives are defined by the needs of others. In the 1980s, there was a spike in writings on codependency, which was seen as contributory to many problems, and as a primary disease in its own right. However, this view did not take hold permanently beyond a milieu of adherents (Mignon, Faiia, Myers, & Rubington, 2009). At the time, individuals who later were diagnosed with problems such as bipolar disorder (manic depression), for example, had chalked up their mood swings to codependency issues. Being the adult child of an alcoholic, it was believed, marked one for long-term, even lifelong emotional problems. More recent research shows that many adult children of alcoholics demonstrate a great deal of resilience and do not necessarily have personality differences from persons growing up in sober families (Burk & Sher, 1990; West & Prinz, 1987; Windle & Searles, 1990).

THE FAMILY ROLE SYSTEM

The family is a system consisting of people playing roles, all of whom have relationships with one another, much as the sun, the planets, and the moons of our solar system exert gravitational and tidal forces on one another and orbit one another. Addiction is a powerful force, and the family role system adapts to it in various ways. If alcoholics neglect their tasks, others must take up the slack. If this responsibility falls to a specific person, that person becomes what family therapist Virginia Satir identified as the superresponsible one (Satir, 1964). Although this person is often the nonalcoholic spouse, tasks may fall to an eldest child, often a female, who was described by Minuchin (1974) as a parental child (sometimes known as a parentified child). A spouse or a parental child may also play the part of rescuer, caretaker, or long-suffering martyr. Another role common in troubled family systems is that of the scapegoat, someone to draw fire, take the blame, and reduce tension. People given that role are often the weakest, the most oddball, or the most problematic. A hyperactive child in an alcoholic family may be scapegoated, even abused. The alcohol abuser himself or herself may be the target, blamed for problems not of his or her making. By scapegoating this person, the family members tells themselves, "If he [or she] didn't drink, we'd be fine" (Edwards, 1990, p. 31).

The family system may factionalize in the presence of alcoholism. A typical constellation is the drinking father and his eldest son as a subsystem against the sober mother and sober children (Edwards, 1990). Or, if the parents both drink, they may constitute a subsystem, with the children left to fend for themselves.

Families can be seen as on a continuum from being overly involved with each other's lives, a condition referred to as being enmeshed, or fused, all the way to being detached, or not having a relationship. It is generally considered healthy for a family to fall somewhere in the middle of this continuum (Minuchin & Fishman, 1981). Families with alcoholism tend to go in either direction, totally circling the wagons, which may entail loss of autonomy and failure to grow as individuals, or they fall apart. The alcoholic may disengage or be thrust out of the family; an eldest child may flee and start his or her own household, which becomes a refuge for others in crisis.

Families in which the alcohol user is recovering have their own problems. A member may have enjoyed some authority or power in the family they otherwise would not have were it not for the alcohol problems. If the adult with an alcohol-use disorder goes through treatment or enters recovery by other means, it may be hard to adjust to the changes that will ensue as the alcohol user becomes assertive and competent, both in terms of adjusting roles and of learning to live with a person with a radically different personality. Statements like "We liked you better drunk" or "Why are you always off at your meetings?" are not uncommon.

It is important to remember that, just each culture has its own language, cuisine, and music, so, too, do family systems, roles, and rules vary tremendously. It is dangerous to assume that there is one kind of family, or one kind of alcoholic family.

HELP FOR FAMILIES WITH ALCOHOL-USE DISORDERS
Al-Anon

Many spouses and significant others of persons with alcohol-use disorders have gotten tremendous support, knowledge, and strength to change by participating in the fellowship of Al-Anon Family Groups. A number of family groups (basically wives' groups) operated independently in the 1940s, and in 1951, Lois Burnham Wilson, the wife of Alcoholics Anonymous founder Bill Wilson, together with her friend Ann B., started a clearinghouse for these groups. This organization became Al-Anon Family Groups, a separate fellowship from AA, although it shares a common philosophy; the Twelve Steps and Twelve Traditions of Al-Anon are based on those of Alcoholics Anonymous. In Al-Anon, family members learn to lovingly detach from the addiction of the member, stop enabling alcoholism, and learn to live their own lives. Alateen is a companion fellowship for young people ages 12–21 (Al-anon, 2011). The principle of "loving detachment" means not making the alcoholic the center of one's life, also called "codependency." This includes:

- not to suffer because of the actions or reactions of other people
- not to allow ourselves to be used or abused by others in the interest of another's recovery
- not to do for others what they could do for themselves
- not to cover up for anyone's mistakes or misdeeds
- not to create a crisis
- not to prevent a crisis if it is in the natural course of events (Al-Anon & Alateen, 2010)

Formal Treatment

Formal treatment agencies often draw in family members for evenings of education about the nature of alcohol-use disorders, enabling, and co-dependent behavior. Extensive family treatment for alcoholism in today's managed-care environment does not get put into practice often outside of expensive private treatment facilities. Nevertheless, such interventions involve but are not limited to

- identifying the system of roles in the family, the investment each person has in his or her role, and the investment others have in their playing this roles
- learning how not to sabotage recovery
- learning how to help the recovering member avoid relapse triggers
- helping facilitate individual growth by practicing healthy communication styles, setting limits, and acknowledging one's feelings and needs

CHAPTER 10

Fetal Alcohol Spectrum Disorders (FASD)

Fetal alcohol spectrum disorders constitute the range of effects that can occur in an individual whose mother drank alcohol during her pregnancy. These effects may include physical, mental, behavioral, and/or learning disabilities with possible lifelong implications. Each year in the United States, as many as 40,000 babies are born with an FASD. Estimates of the costs for FASD alone range from $1 billion to $6 billion a year (Lupton, Burd, & Harwood, 2004).

FASD refers to a spectrum of conditions that include

- fetal alcohol syndrome (FAS)
- fetal alcohol effects (FAE), a milder FASD than full FAS
- alcohol-related neurodevelopmental disorder (ARND)
- alcohol-related birth defects (ARBD)

FASDs occur only when a woman drinks alcohol while pregnant. However, many children prenatally exposed to alcohol are not affected. No safe level of drinking for pregnant women has been determined. The amount of alcohol consumed during pregnancy raises both the risk of FASD and, where it does occur, the severity of FASD. Many FASD fetuses have abnormalities so severe that they spontaneously abort or are stillborn.

CHARACTERISTICS OF CHILDREN WITH FASDs

Physical features of people with fetal alcohol syndrome include a smooth philtrum, the vertical groove between nose and upper lip, and a thin upper lip (see figure 10.1). The face has a flat appearance, including

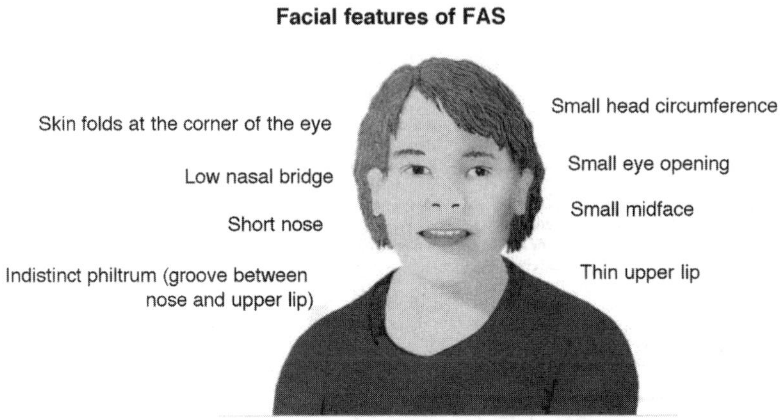

Facial features of FAS

Skin folds at the corner of the eye

Low nasal bridge

Short nose

Indistinct philtrum (groove between nose and upper lip)

Small head circumference

Small eye opening

Small midface

Thin upper lip

Figure 10.1 Craniofacial features associated with fetal alcohol syndrome.

a flat nasal bridge, and eyelids droop and eyes are small and seem to be far apart. The ears appear low set. The child is small and is low in weight before and after birth, and microcephaly occurs, meaning that the head is small, often below the 10th percentile.

With severe FAS, there can also be organ deformities, including heart defects, as well as heart murmurs, genital malformations, and kidney and urinary defects.

The main brain and neurological features of FAS itself include damage to or absence of the corpus callosum, a feature of the brain that contains nerve fibers that bridge the two hemispheres of the brain, as well as damage to the development of the prefrontal cortex (the frontal lobes of the cerebral cortex), abnormal cysts or cavities in the brain, and damage to the development of the basal ganglia.

Neurological/brain abnormalities in FASD can lead to neurological problems, such as seizures, tremors, and poor fine motor skills, and lower-than-average cognitive capacities. Some FASD children can have average intelligence—although many have low normal intelligence and mild or even severe intellectual disabilities—but may have some of the problems listed below. In addition, there are developmental delays in language, social skills, and/or motor skills; learning disabilities, including difficulty in reading or math; difficulty counting money and making change; behavior problems including poor impulse control, which can be misdiagnosed as a conduct disorder; and attention deficit hyperactivity disorder (ADHD). ADHD in a child of high intelligence is not normally associated with an FASD.

The FASD child may have speech and language delays or deficits, poor capacity for abstract thinking, problems in memory or judgment, problems anticipating consequences, difficulty planning or organizing, and difficulty in context-specific learning, or transferring knowledge learned in one situation to another.

The FASD child may have problems in social perception, such as being overly friendly to strangers, being naive, gullible, and easily taken advantage of, having difficultly understanding the perspectives of others, preferring younger friends, and engaging in inappropriate sexual behaviors (Coles & Platzman, 1993; Roebuck, Mattson, & Riley, 1999; Thomas, Kelly, Mattson, & Riley, 1998).

FASD TIMELINE

Amazingly, despite the distinct appearance of persons with severe FASD, it has been studied only since the late 1960s. The term "fetal alcohol syndrome" was first used by Jones and Smith (1973). The term "alcohol embryopathy" was used a few years earlier and continued for some time in the 1970s. In 1988, the U.S. Congress passed the Alcoholic Beverage Labeling Act (see figure 10.2) requiring a health warning statement.

The National Organization on Fetal Alcohol Syndrome was founded in 1990. Awareness of FASD was raised by the publication of *The Broken Cord* (Dorris, 1989), which depicted the difficulties of raising an FASD child. An appreciation of the problems of the moderate-FASD individual came about in the 1990s. These included the so-called secondary disabilities of FASD, social problems that may arise in childhood or teenage years in individuals with an FASD. (Such individuals fare better with early identification and appropriate early interventions.) Secondary disabilities of FASD include disrupted school experiences, trouble with the law, confinement in mental health, substance-abuse treatment, or criminal justice facilities, inappropriate sexual behavior, substance-abuse disorders, and problems with employment (Streissguth, 1994; Streissguth, Barr,

GOVERNMENT WARNING: (1) According to the Surgeon General women should not drink alcoholic beverages during pregnancy because of the risk of birth defects. (2) Consumption of alcoholic beverages impairs your ability to drive a car or operate machinery and may cause health problems.

Figure 10.2 Alcoholic beverage health warning label.

Kogan, & Bookstein, 1996). In 2000, Congress established the FASD Center for Excellence under Section 519D of the Children's Health Act (42 USC 290bb-25d). The center was launched in 2001.

COMMON RISK FACTORS ASSOCIATED WITH HEAVY MATERNAL DRINKING AND FASD

General Features

Aside from heavy maternal drinking per se, poor health of mothers factors into the mix of risk factors, as does the mother being older than 25 when a FAS child is born and having three or more children when a FAS child is born. Other factors include mothers using other drugs, including tobacco and illicit substances, being of an early age at the onset of regular drinking, engaging in frequent binge drinking (i.e., consuming five or more drinks per occasion two or more days per week) and frequent drinking occasions (i.e., every day or every weekend), as well as high blood-alcohol concentration and no reduction in drinking during pregnancy.

Common Features of the Mothers of FASD Children

The mothers of FASD children often have a low socioeconomic status, are socially transient, and are unemployed or marginal employed. They often suffer from depression and low self-esteem, serious mental illnesses, and sexual dysfunction. There is common alcohol misuse in the families of FASD mothers, alcohol misuse by the mother's male partners, lack of marital status, and loss of children to foster or adoptive placement (National Institute on Alcohol Abuse and Alcoholism, 2000; Stratton, Howe, & Battaglia, 1996; May and Gossage, 2001).

FASD EPIDEMIOLOGY

From 0.5 percent to 1.5 percent of children in the United States may suffer from FAS proper, depending on states and communities, and another 1 percent may have milder versions, such as fetal alcohol effect. Native Americans have some of the highest rates of fetal alcohol syndrome in the United States and Canada, but there is considerable variation among groups. The prevalence of FAS among the Navajo, Pueblo Indians, and Southwestern Plains Indians has been studied. Among Southwestern Plains Indians, 10.7 of every 1,000 children were born with FASD, compared with 2.2 per 1,000 for Pueblo Indians and 1.6 for Navajo (May, 1991; May et al., 2000). A spate of media reports in the 1990s quoted alcoholism counselors and writers who claimed that in some communities on reservations, one-fourth of individuals were afflicted with an FASD. South Dakota's Pine Ridge Reservation was especially cited in news reports (NBC News, 2008; *New York Times,* 1990). In contrast, some researchers such as Elizabeth Armstrong and Ernest Abel (Armstrong and Abel, 2000) have asserted that some studies have exaggerated the rates of FASD, and that some FASD campaigning has assumed the status of a moral panic, such as that concerning marijuana in the 1930s or the alleged epidemic of crack babies of the 1980s, which never materialized. Such campaigns, these writers claim, tend to stigmatize lower-income and minority women.

Chudley (2008) points out that many mild FASD cases are surely uncounted. In general, communities where heavy drinking is approved correlate to high rates of FASDs.

Outside of the United States, one of the highest rates of FAS occurs in communities of South Africa. In one Western Cape Province community, 40.5–46.4 per 1,000 children ages 5–9 were diagnosed with the syndrome, and age-specific community rates for ages 6–7 were 39.2–42.9 (Centers for Disease Control and Prevention, 2003; May et al., 2000).

In 2010, following the return of an adopted child to Russia by parents who claimed he was behaviorally unmanageable, public attention was also focused on the high rates of FASDs among children in Russian orphanages (Belluck, 2010), a phenomenon already well known to researchers. One study of children in a Murmansk, Russia, orphanage found 45 percent of children with some fetal alcohol effect and 15 percent with full-fledged FAS (Miller et al., 2006).

CHAPTER 11

Treatment and Recovery

Recovery is a self-directed, ongoing process by which individuals attain sobriety, get their lives under control, manage them effectively, and move in the direction of emotional, behavioral, interpersonal, and cognitive health. Abstaining from the abuse of alcohol and other drugs is necessary but not sufficient for a full recovery from a substance-use disorder. Recovery may involve episodes of professional treatment and/or participation in mutual aid fellowships or religion. Recovery movements, and their role in the beginnings of alcohol treatment, are discussed in the first part of this chapter.

Treatment is a set of formal, professional, science-based interventions and services that offer skills and tools for initiating and maintaining recovery, and facilitate movement through stages of change toward a full recovery. These are outlined in the second part of this chapter.

RECOVERY MOVEMENTS AND BEGINNINGS OF ALCOHOL TREATMENT

Roots of Recovery Movements

Movements for recovery from alcohol problems are deeply rooted in American culture. Grassroots voluntary associations of all sorts are an American phenomenon, noted as far back as 1835 by Alexis de Tocqueville (De Tocqueville, 2000). Popular health and mental health movements, often with a religious or spiritual emphasis, have flourished in America for over 150 years (Engs, 2000).

Temperance movements in particular have come and gone since the early 19th century. At that time, temperance was part of the platform of the emerging African American church denominations and of the abolitionist movement, not as a moral issue but as one of health and self-determination. Later, temperance was part of the suffragist movement. In addition to the many temperance and prohibition groups such as the Woman's Christian Temperance Union and the Anti-Saloon League came self-help associations of reformed drunks such as the Washingtonians, who at one point in the mid-19th century had 100,000 adherents (Blumberg & Pittman, 1991). The United Order of Ex-Boozers was another example of such formations during the century before Alcoholics Anonymous was founded. Finally, religious organizations such as the Salvation Army, as well as homeless missions, targeted alcoholics in particular.

Temperance and prohibition movements had tremendous impact in the first two decades of the 20th century. County by county, state by state, the nation went dry, culminating in the passage of the 19th Amendment in 1919, establishing national Prohibition, and implemented via the Volstead Act. The amendment was repealed in 1933, two years before the founding of Alcoholics Anonymous.

The immediate predecessor of Alcoholics Anonymous was the Oxford Group, a middle-class evangelical Protestant group flourishing in the early 1930s led by Frank Buchman. It sought to emulate the intimacy of early, first-century Christianity by organizing small group meetings that focused on five Procedures: Give in to God, Follow God's Direction, Check Guidance, Restitution, and Sharing for Witness and for Confession. Alcoholics were a particular target of the Oxford Group's efforts (Kurtz, 1998), particularly in Akron, Ohio.

Alcoholics Anonymous

In June 1935, two alcoholic members of the Oxford Group, William Griffiths Wilson (the famous Bill W.) and Robert Smith (Dr. Bob) were introduced in Akron, Ohio. They formed the nucleus of an alcoholic wing of the Oxford Group that peeled off and developed its own fellowship in 1937–1939. To a large extent, AA adapted the program of the Oxford Group for alcoholics but also was influenced by William James, who saw religious conversion as a prerequisite for recovery from alcoholism, and by C. J. Jung, who had a similar viewpoint. The basic text of AA, simply titled *Alcoholics Anonymous* but known as the Big Book, was written in 1939. The latest edition is 1976 (Alcoholics Anonymous, 1976). It is available to read or download online (http//:www.aa.org/bigbookonline/).

AA is a democratic, grassroots fellowship or mutual-aid society of people wishing to achieve sobriety from alcohol. It has been described as a source of folk psychotherapy or a grassroots therapeutic social movement, as opposed to a professional or academically based school of psychotherapy or treatment (Alibrandi, 1985). AA is fiercely independent of social and medical institutions.

It is founded on the principle of anonymity; first names and initials of surnames are used (as with the use of "Bill W." for the founder). Its internal structure is also unusual in that it is completely democratic, unstratified, and nonhierarchical.

The AA method is based on the Twelve Steps (which can be read at http://www.aa.org/en_pdfs/smf-121_en.pdf), and its basic organizational posture is based on the Twelve Traditions (which can be read at http://www.aa.org/pdf/products/p-43_thetwelvetradiillustrated.pdf). Recovery consists of working the steps in order. The final step involves reaching out to other alcoholics and spreading the recovery message.

Many principles and methods of AA involve a so-called Higher Power, a spiritual concept left deliberately nonspecific in order to appeal to a wide variety of people and to avoid the appearance of AA as an organized religion. Frequent attendance at AA meetings is strongly suggested, at which members tell their story of decline due to drinking, a spiritual awakening, and their lives after alcohol. Attending 90 meetings in 90 days after quitting alcohol is encouraged. Members never consider themselves cured, but refer to themselves as recovering, basically in remission from alcoholism, one day at a time. Membership in AA is lifelong, and total abstinence is required to be in recovery.

The philosophy of AA is boiled down into mottoes that are clear, concrete, and understandable to newly sober or barely sober alcoholics: "One Day at a Time," "Don't Drink and Go to Meetings," and "Let Go and Let God." AA's World Service Office publishes extensive literature, and there is a great emphasis on reading these works. The books alone, many of which concerns the early history and evolution of AA and the nature of the disease of alcoholism, will fill an entire bookshelf.

AA policy states that alcoholism is a lifelong, chronic, and progressive disease and that one must be continually vigilant about the possibilities of relapse. In this philosophy, it prefigured the standard model of alcoholic disease found outside of AA in alcoholism treatment and in the medical community at large.

AA provides strong group cohesion and group affiliation, catharsis, conversion to a sober ideology, and a sober subculture within which to live (Emrick, 1987; Kassel & Wagner, 1993). What goes on after and between meetings is crucial; members stay in touch with each other and with their sponsor, a kind of big brother or mentor who keeps track of his or her "sponsee." Meetings are available throughout the day in many places. Although no precise census is available, the fellowship numbers about five million members.

For decades following the founding of AA, it remained the only place where alcoholics could go and get help. There was deep distrust between AA and the medical institutions, which alcoholics felt had been of little help to them in their suffering. Conversely, these institutions had little respect for the capabilities of untrained, recovering alcoholics to treat any behavioral-health issue. The basic template and model of AA has spawned many spin-offs and similar groups, known in general as 12-step groups. The largest of these are Narcotics Anonymous and Gamblers Anonymous, but 12-step groups exist in the worlds of eating disorders, sexual disorders, and various other compulsions and social problems such as indebtedness.

Alternatives to Alcoholics Anonymous

SMART Recovery (the acronym is from "Self Management and Recovery Training"), which is not a spiritual program and does not consider alcoholism to be a disease, is the best-known alternative to AA. It does not intend membership to be a lifelong affair, as with AA. It was originally based on the concept of rational emotive behavior therapy developed by Albert Ellis (Ellis, McInerney, DiGiuseppe, & Yeager, 1988), but it has incorporated other contemporary addiction-treatment models such as the Stages of Change model (described later in this section) and cognitive-behavioral techniques for relapse prevention. Face-to-face and online meetings are available. In some parts of the United States, meetings are sparse, but the program has caught on in certain cities such as Tucson, Arizona, and San Diego, California. Some of the core features of the program include that it

- involves teaching self-empowerment and self-reliance
- works on addictions and compulsions as complex maladaptive behaviors with possible physiological factors
- includes teaching tools and techniques for self-directed change
- encourages individuals to recover and live satisfying lives
- includes meetings that are educational and include open discussions
- advocates the appropriate use of prescribed medications and psychological treatments
- evolves as scientific knowledge evolves, as opposed to an unchanging dogma or philosophy
- differs from Alcoholics Anonymous, Narcotics Anonymous, and traditional 12-step programs

Meetings can be located at their main Web site: http://www.smartrecov
ery.org.

The tools and techniques of SMART Recovery may be downloaded
from http://www.smartrecovery.org/resources/toolchest.htm. The purposes
and methods of SMART Recovery are detailed in the appendices.

Secular Organizations for Sobriety (SOS), also known as Save Our
Selves, was started by Jim Christopher in 1985 as a secular-humanist alternative to AA. It is abstinence based and, like AA, considers alcoholism a disease but maintains a secular approach as opposed to a spiritual
outlook. Christopher remains executive director a quarter-century later
(Christopher, 1988, 1989). SOS exists in all states of the United States
but most chapters are in California, New York, and Texas. It promotes a
straightforward program for avoiding relapse comparable both to that of
AA and cognitive-behavioral therapy, and daily acknowledgment of the
alcohol problem is emphasized. SOS presents two concepts, a Cycle of
Addiction and a Cycle of Sobriety, that mirror, in a less technical fashion,
some of our understandings of addictions and recovery motivation today.
SOS meetings can be located at the organization's main Web site, http://
www.sossobriety.org.

Founded in 2001, LifeRing is a spin-off from SOS. LifeRing found-
ers wished to be independent of the secular humanist tradition. LifeRing
members may utilize various methods they find useful. More information
can be found on their main Web site: http://lifering.org/.

The 16-Step Program is based on the work of Charlotte Kasl, who modified the 12 steps, which she felt were extremely out of date. She imported
a feminist perspective, substituted empowerment for powerlessness, and
toned down the Higher Power perspective found in the 12 Step model. Kasl
borrows from various spiritual traditions including Zen and Quaker perspectives, positive psychology, and resilience theory. According to Kasl,
there are now well over 200 face-to-face recovery support groups based on
this model. More information can be found on their main Web site: http://
www.charlottekasl.com/site/16-step-program.

Women for Sobriety (WFS) was founded by Jean Kirkpatrick in 1976
to serve the special recovery needs of women. Kirkpatrick, a sociologist,
had been active in AA but found it did not meet her needs. The program is
founded on its Statement of Purpose and Thirteen Affirmations. Although
the founder is now deceased, the program continues to operate in many
states. Basic principles of WFS and meetings can be located by contacting
the organization at http://www.womenforsobriety.org.

Moderation Management (MM), a radical departure from AA or any
of its secular alternatives, is a self-help organization supporting problem

drinkers in their attempt to cut down to a moderate, responsible level of drinking. The controversy over this approach is discussed under Key Issues and Controversies, below, and the principles of MM are detailed in the appendices. Opponents of the MM program consider a moderation program as a form of Russian roulette, as no one can know for sure who can successfully moderate and who will simply fall back into a severe alcohol-use disorder by not staying away from alcohol entirely. More information as well as contact information is available at http://www.moderation.org.

EMERGENCE OF ALCOHOLISM TREATMENT

In early AA, members, including Bill W., filled their houses with people trying to get and stay dry. They established AA clubhouses, homes, and retreats, and they worked as volunteers in hospitals, reaching out to alcoholics. Some of these activities evolved into a more structured form intermediate between AA proper and real, institutionalized treatment programs (Yalisove, 1998). Eventually, formal programs emerged, largely staffed by AA members and following AA philosophy that was the basis for the alcoholism-treatment community. Specialized hospitals to treat alcoholism had come and gone during the first half of the 20th century. In fact, Bill W., the cofounder of Alcoholics Anonymous, had a dramatic spiritual-conversion experience in New York City's Towns Hospital, when he began his sobriety. However, true inpatient rehabilitation facilities, or rehabs, arose in Minnesota during the 1950s. They included patient education through didactic groups and AA meetings, and then added assessment-based treatment planning (from social work) and individual and group counseling, and began to hire professionals as well to form interdisciplinary treatment teams. Oddly, the length of stay in rehab was almost invariably 28 days, a number that was a response to insurance-coverage limitations in Minnesota but had no valid basis as a treatment period. Nevertheless, the 28-day stay became an industry standard. Some state hospitals established alcoholism units along these lines in the early 1960s. States and municipalities, as well as AA members, also set up so-called drying-out or sobering-up stations or detoxification units in the late 1960s and early 1970s. AA had allies in the professional world, including E. M. Jellinek, who detailed the disease concept of alcoholism and its separate species, as he called them. In the 1940s, Jellinek established the Yale School of Alcohol Studies and the Yale Plan Clinics, the first modern outpatient treatment program for alcoholics. He also supported AA member Marty Mann in forming the National Council on Alcoholism, which championed the public acceptance of alcoholism as a disease and was a bridge to the scientific and professional community.

Rehabs proliferated in the 1970s, but the real heyday of such facilities was in the 1980s, when expensive private facilities flourished and insurance companies paid blindly for what they were billed. This is now seen as an era of excess for which the treatment community paid dearly.

Also noteworthy is the fact that alcoholism counselors were by and large nondegreed paraprofessionals who themselves were in recovery from alcoholism. There were no systems for accrediting counselors until the late 1970s, and when these systems were constructed, at their onset they rarely had a substantial educational requirement. In addition, not only was alcoholism treatment separate from mental health treatment, but most states also had separate state authorities for alcohol abuse and for drug problems, and when counselor credentialing arose, many states had separate credentials for alcoholism counselors and drug counselors, and separate accreditation boards.

With the advent of managed care, third-party payers were less and less likely to pay for inpatient stays lasting weeks. At the same time, researchers (Hayashida et al., 1989) challenged the rationale for inpatient care as a standard method for treating alcoholism. Well over half of inpatient facilities have closed over the past 20 years, and lengths of stay have declined in the remainder. Between 1994 and 1997 alone, 67 percent of inpatient substance-abuse programs offered by the Department of Veterans Affairs closed, leaving only programs for veterans with co-occurring mental illnesses in addiction to substance abuse (Humphreys, Huebsch, Moos, & Suchinsky, 1999).

ELEMENTS OF TREATMENT FOR ALCOHOL-USE DISORDERS
How and Why People Enter Treatment

Treatment for alcohol-use problems and disorders is initiated by some mixture of desperation, compulsion, and natural desires to achieve health. Often, all three are needed.

Desperation

Chronic alcohol abusers or alcoholics experience problems with some or all aspects of their lives, including job, school, family members, the law, and their own body. As we detailed in Part 1, they are caught up in a vicious, worsening spiral of problems and pain. Alcoholics Anonymous has the concept of hitting bottom, which in the early days of AA meant homelessness, jail, or severe physical illness. But the bottom, a point beyond which a person just can't stand his or her situation, might be much less desperate. A member of AA, a successful lawyer and a functional alcoholic, recounted his bottom: A wake-up call came when a taxi driver asked whether he was all right, and when the passenger asked why, the driver said, "Because you're drunk."

Compulsion

However horribly alcohol users may feel, they usually need a push to get involved with treatment. Family members may become fed up with their out-of-control alcohol-use behaviors and demand that they get help. Employers, schools, and other institutions and organizations have mechanisms to identify and refer persons with alcohol problems and disorders into treatment. Many of the institutions in the list have developed formal linkages with treatment programs, which may assess and refer clients to the appropriate level of care and treatment modality matching their problem, or may provide the treatment themselves.

Employers have employee-assistance programs, or EAPs. Unions have member-assistance programs, and schools and school districts may have student-assistance programs, or SAPs. (These terms are polite ways of referring to substance-abuse screening and referral programs.) Child-welfare and welfare-to-work programs have increasingly implemented substance-abuse referral programs, which greatly improve their success. Courts and criminal justice systems have increasingly implemented alternatives to incarceration options for persons whose lawbreaking was substance related. States have recognized that recidivism is greatly reduced when treatment options are offered.

Natural Recovery

Health aspirations and motives are present in even the most severe substance abuser. Many people stop or moderate drinking of their own accord, or via affiliation or reaffiliation with a religious institution. Movement out of an alcohol-abusing subculture may facilitate maturing out, as when a heavy-drinking member of an unregulated campus fraternity moderates or ceases drinking upon graduation. For some, an engagement or a marriage, the arrival of a new child, or the possibility of a job may be a stake in moving into recovery.

Screening and Referral for Alcohol-Use Disorders

It is recommended that all medical-care, social services, and even dental-care providers use simple screening techniques to identify whether clients have an alcohol-use disorder. In practice, it does not take place that often, a fact the reader can verify by trying to recall when one's physician asked them about one's drinking. A number of simple screening instruments are available online from the Center for Substance Abuse Treatment (1995).

Also, government agencies can screen for alcohol-use disorders to determine whether a client is eligible and appropriate for receiving agency services. Eligibility might concern the client's insurance coverage or his or her age, appropriateness might concern whether a client stands to succeed at that particular facility or needs specialized services such as a gay-friendly atmosphere, an interpreter, or a staff familiar with, say, disabilities and alcoholism.

Screening should also identify the person's level of severity and should prompt referral into an appropriate level of care. Following the insurance backlash against treatments for alcoholism, many plans allowed for only five days of treatment or less. The American Society for Addiction Medicine (2001) promulgated a rational system to determine the level of severity of addiction symptoms, which constitute criteria for placement into different levels of care and show a sound medical basis for the provision of treatment. ASAM uses six dimensions in its Patient Placement Criteria to assess the severity of addiction: Acute-withdrawal potential, medical conditions and complications, psychiatric conditions or complications, readiness to change, relapse potential, and recovery environment. The individual is rated from 1 to 4 on all six dimensions. A more complete description of the six dimensions is presented in Appendix A (pp. 191–193). Depending on the level of severity, the individual is referred to or placed in an appropriate level of care, also according to a model devised by ASAM, which to put it most simply, is outpatient, intensive outpatient, and inpatient café. (See the next section.)

If the individual is physically addicted to alcohol and is likely to suffer severe withdrawal symptoms, he or she may need to be medically stabilized in what may be called a detoxification or medical-stabilization unit, or, colloquially, detox. Detoxification consists of ridding the system of alcohol while attending to medical needs during the acute-withdrawal phase., which may include the use of antiseizure or antianxiety drugs and monitoring of vital signs. The length of stay is usually three to five days. There was, and continues to be, considerable confusion about detox: One hears statements such as, "My brother-in-law John went through detox six times, and he still drinks," supposedly testifying to the failure of alcoholism treatment. Detoxification is merely medical stabilization and the precursor to treatment. Considerable care is needed to make sure that John isn't back out on the street, but rather goes directly into a rehabilitation program. The patient may be willing to enter detoxification because he or she feels simply awful, but after detoxification, an alcoholic will feel better, and his or her fears about participating in extended treatment will predominate, and the person may vacillate or refuse to continue. Detoxification also takes place on an outpatient basis for milder forms of alcoholism, which would have been unheard of until the 1990s (Hayashida et al., 1989).

Levels of Care

The basic levels of care formulated by ASAM include the following (Center for Substance Abuse Treatment, 1993):

Level 0.5: Early intervention for at-risk individuals without a diagnosis of alcohol-use disorder.

Level I: Outpatient services, including evaluation, treatment, and recovery management, all on a nonresidential basis, from one to ten hours per week. In fact, outpatient services can perform several functions:

Comprehensive treatment for an alcohol-use disorder without removing an individual from work or school, thereby not disrupting the person's occupational or educational status.

An initial point of contact for the individual who may be a walk-in or a referral from a family member or a law-enforcement agency familiar with this particular program. The client may then be assessed and sent to a more rigorous level of care, such as one described below.

An after-care facility for an individual who has been discharged on completion of an inpatient rehabilitation stay.

Outpatient detoxification.

Level II: Intensive outpatient treatment (II.1) and partial hospitalization services (II.5), which clients can attend after work or school. They may reside at home or in a long-term-care facility, in a special apartment program, or in some other form of therapeutic residence. Again, this treatment avoids disrupting normal life, promotes bonding among members of the program, and costs at least half of residential care. Also, participants can apply their new skills to real-world environments while in treatment.

Level III: Residential/inpatient services can be managed by nonmedical personnel, but can also be medically monitored. Inpatient services can be rehabilitative or can be provided in a nonmedical detoxification facility.

Level IV: Medically managed intensive inpatient services in a hospital or a medical center when a person needs 24-hour treatment and medical, nursing, or psychiatric care or a combination thereof. Medical problems such were outlined in previous sections, pertaining to alcohol effects on the liver, the pancreas, the brain, and so on, will be addressed at this level. This medical setting can be a rehabilitation facility that provides the services of medical and psychiatric social workers and credentialed alcoholism counselors during a three- or four-week stay. Short-term hospital-based detoxification also falls within this level.

Assessment and Treatment Planning

Assessment is the gathering of information from many sources, including self-reporting, about a range of areas, usually including:

Childhood and adolescent history
History of clients' alcohol use and abuse
Health problems and medical history, past and present
Mental health history
Family and social functioning
Employment and educational history
Sexual history
Financial status
Legal issues
Assessment of severity
Assessment of readiness to change (see the Stages of Change paradigm further on in this chapter)

Based on the information gathered in assessment, the client and his or her counselor work together to plan for how the client may be helped by participation in the services provided by an agency or program. This is a collaborative effort to identify:

Issues, problems, and needs
Strengths and supports
Readiness to change in each problem area
Long-term goals
Specific short-term objectives toward attaining these goals
Criteria for monitoring whether objectives are being met
Services and methods needed to help the client meet objectives

A plan for discharge into the posttreatment world to ensure that supports are in place to help in continued and strengthened sobriety

WHAT HAPPENS IN TREATMENT

Alcoholism treatment differs from conventional counseling in that its consumers are, with the exception of persons with serious mental illnesses, typically more deteriorated medically, psychologically, and socially than run-of-the-mill counseling clients. Because of these factors, treatment tends to be more structured and directive, as well as more comprehensive in scope. Moreover, because serious alcoholism is a life-threatening condition, counseling and treatment make it a priority to get clients medically, psychologically, and socially stabilized. These goals involve concrete and simple objectives involving here-and-now situations. Discussions about past events take a back burner to the achievement of a steady sobriety, tools to avoid relapse, and considerations about legal and medical concerns.

Individual Counseling

Just as in ordinary psychotherapy, a variety of models and methods exist to choose from, but most modern alcoholism counselors have an eclectic model that synthesizes the best approaches from all fields and methods. The specific school or theory of counseling is less important than the priority of building a collaborative, empathetic relationship between counselor and client. Individual counseling usually addresses feelings (affects), behavior, and thinking (cognition) and how they interrelate, as well as interpersonal issues such as the following:

- Emotions: Alcohol abusers or alcoholics have often suppressed or numbed their feelings with chemical anesthesia. When they are newly sober, feelings may come pouring out and frighten them. They need to be able to identify their emotions, assertively and appropriately communicate them, and not be fearful or guilty about them. They need to know that being angry, for example, does not have to be associated with violence or destructiveness, as it is when they are drunk. They have to learn to talk about feelings rather than drink about them.
- Behavior: Alcohol abusers are often used to living in chaos, disorganization, hopelessness, and defeat. Learning how to be responsible is an important step toward a real recovery. Alcoholics also need to avoid triggers for relapse, an idea Alcoholics Anonymous sums up in

the motto "Stay away from people, places, and things" (that remind you or tempt you to drink).

- Thinking: Cognitive and cognitive-behavioral psychologists (Beck, Wright, Newman, & Liese, 1993; Ellis et al., 1988) have described irrational ways of thinking that make people miserable and also prone to drink. Awfulizing, or catastrophizing, is one example of a way of thinking that magnifies the significance of a trivial setback into a nightmare of anxiety that would prompt drinking. Beliefs like "I can't get through the day without a drink" or "I can't have fun without drinking" or "I can't talk to girls without drinking" trigger cravings.
- Interpersonal realm: There are many areas in which people recovering from an alcohol-use disorder need to work on interpersonal relationships: They may have socialized only with other heavy drinkers and in bars. They will need to develop sober relationships. They may have to learn to communicate and interact with others while sober, and without the crutch of alcohol.

As described in the section on alcohol and the family, families often adapt in an unhealthy way around the addiction. Patterns of denial, concealment, enabling, and codependency may need years of undoing. Worse, family members may have been rejected by, or may have removed themselves out of shame from, family and social networks. Sober sexuality may be an unknown, and may raise significant anxiety.

The communication style of a person recovering from an alcohol-use disorder probably requires a major overhaul. There may have been destructive patterns of communication, dishonesty, withdrawal, and hostility and aggression, as opposed to an open, honest, appropriate, and assertive mode of communication.

Group Counseling

Most alcoholism treatment takes place in groups. These groups break down the social and emotional isolation of alcoholics, provide valuable role models, and help participants realize that others in the group share most of their problems and secrets, which reduces guilt and anxiety. They provide practice in communicating emotion. Clients enjoy groups. Also, groups are, importantly, very cost effective. The kinds of groups that behavioral-health and addictions treatment provide is different in format from those in Alcoholics Anonymous. AA meetings have a more round-robin approach, in which people take turns telling their stories, and cross-talk is discouraged. In groups such as are common in mental-health and alcoholism settings, however, interaction is the whole idea of the group. Various group settings include the following:

- As opposed to treatment groups per se, alcoholism facilities have a range of classroom-style presentations and discussions of issues pertaining to alcohol and alcoholism itself, treatment and recovery issues, and special issues such as sexuality or anger.
- Alcoholism counselors assist with case management and coordination of services with the courts, medical facilities, housing and homeless services, entitlement programs, and vocational-educational services for alcoholics.
- It is important for the significant others of the recovering alcoholic to be brought in to be educated on the nature of alcohol-use disorders, to show them what the client is going through as they enter recovery, to prepare them for the newly recovering family member and help them resist undermining recovery or engaging in behavior that enables a relapse, and in avoiding going over past grievances and grudges.

DISCHARGE PLANNING

A long-term recovery plan is needed following formal treatment. The alcoholic may be going back to the same environment that contributed to or enabled alcohol abuse. This issue is addressed later in the section on long-term-recovery support. Housing needs, placement into a vocational and educational system, and ongoing medical services should be addressed. But not everyone is ready to go back into the community, and other alternatives exist.

Reentry residences, halfway houses, recovery houses, and cooperative living arrangements are supportive, therapeutic environments for the individual discharged from residential treatment but needing a step-down residence before transitioning back into the community. Halfway houses often have a work requirement and may involve an element of client self-government. Notable in this regard are Oxford Houses, which are democratically operated and self-supported, voting to elect officers and admit members. Oxford Houses are a tremendous resource for maintenance of long-term recovery (Jason & Ferrari, 2009; Jason, Olson, & Foli, 2008). Over 1,000 sober residences use the Oxford House (2011) model.

Long-term-care residential facilities such as those run by the Salvation Army and Goodwill Industries serve individuals incapable of independent living. They amount to a structured shelter situation, often with a work component; counseling services are often offered. Supportive apartment programs are maintained by social-services agencies for alcoholics who have co-occurring psychiatric disorders.

CONFIDENTIALITY

Alcoholism treatment, like all behavioral-health treatment, is governed by strict federal and state guidelines that forbid release of information without the express written consent of the patient. The counseling relationship exists in a cone of silence and privacy like that of an attorney and client. The staff and administration of alcoholism-treatment facilities are bound to go to great effort to ensure privacy and confidentiality of patient information, changing computer passwords, ensuring that they log off from a computer if they leave it, and even insuring that a passing person cannot see what is on a computer screen. It is not within the scope of this volume to list all of the statutes within the Code of Federal Regulations Title 42 (CFR 42) and Health Insurance Portability and Accountability Act (HIPAA) regulations, which are summarized to the client at the point of intake into the agency.

TRENDS IN ALCOHOL TREATMENT IN THE SECOND DECADE OF THE 21ST CENTURY

Alcoholism treatment is still in transition from older traditional models to evidence-based treatment. It is difficult to evaluate what treatment methods are based on evidence, because almost any counseling effort is productive, people who enter and complete treatment are already demonstrating momentum and motivation to heal, and many people remit spontaneously from addictive disorders. Moreover, therapeutic relationships are more important than the particular school of treatment employed. A few of the 21st-century trends are presented in this section. None of these models need be in conflict with active membership in Alcoholics Anonymous. It should be borne in mind, as well, that a majority of people with alcohol-use disorders experience at least one relapse before recovering.

The Transtheoretical Stages of Change model is based on the work of Prochaska and DiClemente (1982), who observed that healthy change involved several stages, processes, and tasks (see also Prochaska, Norcross, & DiClemente, 1994). Their observations were of people who gave up smoking tobacco on their own, but these have been extrapolated as useful in many addictive and other health-decision areas. The stages are as follows:

Precontemplation (not thinking about changing)—The person may be resisting or denying change, may be in despair, or both. The person might be leveraged into treatment, however.

Contemplation (thinking about changing)—The person sees that he or she has a problem but is not ready to change or even to prepare to change.

Preparing to change—This stage involves some commitment or anticipation of action, but there is a great deal of ambivalence, and the person may fall back from this stage.

Action stage—This stage involves real behavioral change and beginning healthy behaviors.

Maintenance stage—This stage involves consolidating and strengthening the gains made in the action stage.

Termination stage—In this stage, the person has moved past the problem-solving stages entirely. (A person familiar with the Alcoholics Anonymous philosophy might worry about defining oneself as being in this stage, as alcoholics, according to AA, recover one day at a time, and thinking that one is an ex-alcoholic would be considered putting oneself in danger.)

Almost no one moves right through these stages; the model is one of an upward spiral, and one falls back into an earlier stage and then moves forward again. This progress is seen as a normal part of the cycles of growth (Prochaska et al., 1994). The counselor's role is to facilitate movement through the stages of change. This is an ambitious and optimistic view of the alcohol abuser, recognizing that they have strengths, desires and ambitions to be rid of their affliction.

Assessment of readiness to change involves figuring out the pluses and minuses of change in the mind of the drinker. This can involve a decisional balance sheet, a tool that was originally proposed by Irving Janis and Leo Mann (1977) for smoking-cessation therapy. Here, we have substituted alcohol-related items:

Benefits of changing	Benefits of not changing
I'll feel better	Why change? It's easier to stay the same
I'll keep my job	It's fun to drink
My family will be happy	This way, I don't have to feel the bad stuff

Downside of changing	Downside of not changing
I'll go into withdrawal again good	My wife will finally throw me out for
I won't be able to sleep	I'll ruin my liver and die
If I fail, I'll really be in despair	I'll get more DWIs and lose my license

Velasquez, Maurer, Crouch, and DiClemente (2001) recommend rating each item from 1 to 4 as slightly, moderately, very, or extremely important. Even when at the very beginning of treatment, this assessment of motives has the healthy effect of sorting out motives, and, in fact, moves the client into contemplating change. What it shows us, in addition, is that the alcohol user is very ambivalent about his or her behavior, as opposed to the common view that he or she was simply in denial and then miraculously catapulted into recovery.

A newer, cognitive-behavioral relapse-prevention model that dovetails with the upward spiral of the Stages of Change is that of Alan Marlatt (Marlatt & Donovan, 2008). Originally proposed in 1985, it has caught on over the past decade and a half as an alternative to the model of all-or-nothing recovery versus relapse.

According to Marlatt, black-and-white thinking about recovery can turn a minor slip into a total severe relapse. Having a drink, under the black/white dichotomy, signals failure and gives permission to proceed into a bender. Marlatt says that having a drink is an error, not a defeat, and moreover, provides a teachable moment that can contribute to continued progress in recovery by figuring out how the person could handle things better the next time a temptation is presented. Larimer, Palmer, & Marlatt (1999) offer an extensive overview of the Marlatt model.

Classic alcoholism treatment saw the client as in massive denial. This view, in fact, was a cornerstone of the disease concept of alcoholism. But as we just saw above, there are all sorts of pluses and minuses rattling around in the head of the drinker. Miller and Rollnick (1991), who pioneered new thinking about the motives of drinkers, stated that ambivalence is natural, fluctuating, and ongoing before, during and after treatment. Their method, which is also tied into the Stages of Change model just described, is known as motivational interviewing, or motivational-enhancement therapy. In contrast to classic alcoholism treatment, MI does not confront individuals to break through denial and hit them with labels like *addict*. Confrontation and labeling is seen as a trap that promotes resistance and denial behaviors. Rather, it works with people at whatever level in the Stages of Change they may be. It avoids argumentation and is empathic, accepting, and respectful.

At the same time, it develops discrepancies between drinkers' current behavior and their broader goals, and supports self-efficacy. A synthesis of research on MI (Burke, Arkowitz, & Menchola, 2003) concludes that it an effective model.

It is not within the scope of this volume to provide a complete outline of MI, but further information is available at http://www.motivationalinter view.org and http://casaa.unm.edu/manuals/met.pdf.

Working with motives is only one part of the equation. The counseling package includes mobilizing intervention pressures and leveraging a person to get into and stay in treatment, providing incentives, working with the person's family to remove enabling, and providing case management to ensure that the client has basics like a place to stay.

It's paradoxical that although it has long been stated that alcoholism is a chronic and relapsing condition, treatment more resembles acute care, as if it were a strep throat infection. Research clearly shows that successful recovery doesn't rest on the methods or intensity of what goes on the relatively short, formal treatment episode as much as it does on continuous, long-term support, even on an inexpensive and low level (McClellan, 2002). Extended case monitoring is shown to be cost effective (Stout, Rubin, Zwick, Zywiak, & Bellino, 1999). To this end, a number of recovery-support initiatives have arisen, including simple telephone monitoring of people in recovery, often by minimally trained recovery mentors, recovery coaches, or peer wellness specialists. A comprehensive series of monographs and papers on peer-recovery support is available at http://www.attcnetwork.org/regcenters/ c2.asp?rcid=3&content=CUSTOM2.

While the redemptive themes of alcoholic recovery have been a theme in American culture for 200 years, they long mainly stayed within the self-help and religious milieus. Around the turn of the millennium, however, public advocacy for the reduction of stigma, support for treatment and research, and celebration of recovery became a national social movement. A national coalition of individuals and organizations, Faces and Voices of Recovery (FVR), was founded in 2001. On its Web site, each member of the board of FVR lists the year in which he or she entered recovery. In addition, various prominent public figures proclaimed their recovery status and their championing of recovery support. In 2004, the Congressional Addiction, Treatment, and Recovery Caucus was formed under the leadership of U.S. representatives Patrick Kennedy (D-RI) and Jim Ramstad (R-MN). Kennedy and Ramstad introduced the Paul Wellstone Mental Health and Addiction Equity Act, which was voted into law in 2008 with widespread lobbying support by FVR.

As part of this public-recovery trend, recovery from alcohol abuse and alcoholism has become the subject of many autobiographies, a subset of memoirs of illness and dysfunction, a major genre in American writing of the late 20th and early 21st centuries. Augusten Burroughs (2003), Susan Cheever (1999), Pete Hamill (1994), Carolyn Knapp (1996), and Neil Steinberg (1999) are some of the prominent authors who have chronicled their years of drinking and stopping drinking.

The U.S. government's Substance Abuse and Mental Health Administration has championed Screening, Brief Intervention, and Referral to Treatment (SBIRT), a specific form of brief intervention demonstrated to have produced positive results in early intervention with alcohol abusers. Over a half a million individuals have been screened at trauma centers and emergency rooms, community clinics, federally qualified health centers, and school clinics. Some of the specific screening instruments are presented in Appendix A. The core components of SBIRT can be defined as shown in figure 11.1.

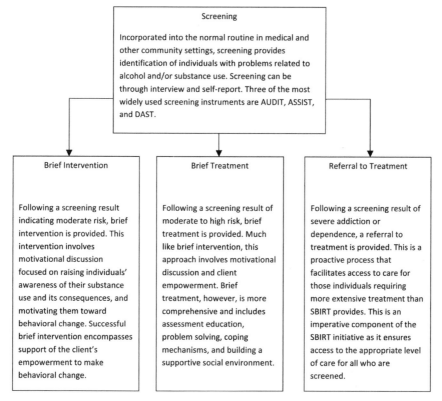

Screening

Incorporated into the normal routine in medical and other community settings, screening provides identification of individuals with problems related to alcohol and/or substance use. Screening can be through interview and self-report. Three of the most widely used screening instruments are AUDIT, ASSIST, and DAST.

Brief Intervention

Following a screening result indicating moderate risk, brief intervention is provided. This intervention involves motivational discussion focused on raising individuals' awareness of their substance use and its consequences, and motivating them toward behavioral change. Successful brief intervention encompasses support of the client's empowerment to make behavioral change.

Brief Treatment

Following a screening result of moderate to high risk, brief treatment is provided. Much like brief intervention, this approach involves motivational discussion and client empowerment. Brief treatment, however, is more comprehensive and includes assessment education, problem solving, coping mechanisms, and building a supportive social environment.

Referral to Treatment

Following a screening result of severe addiction or dependence, a referral to treatment is provided. This is a proactive process that facilitates access to care for those individuals requiring more extensive treatment than SBIRT provides. This is an imperative component of the SBIRT initiative as it ensures access to the appropriate level of care for all who are screened.

Figure 11.1   SBIRT: Core components.

Preliminary research on SBIRT in the United States shows that it decreases the frequency and severity of alcohol misuse, reduces the risk of trauma, and increases enrollment in specialized alcohol-abuse treatment (Babor et al., 2007). Some public-health researchers feel, in fact, that brief interventions have more effect, dollar for dollar, than costly, formal treatment programs (Wutzke, Conigrave, Saunders, & Hall, 2002). Other studies (Roche & Freeman, 2004), however, have found that, if one examines brief interventions on an international scale, they are hobbled by physicians' fear that they will lose patients, physician disinterest in alcohol problems, lack of time, and lack of skill in administering the screening instruments. It may be uncomfortable for a physician or another helping professional to suddenly hit a person with a formal questionnaire. In fact, one study (Vinson, Galliher, Reidinger, & Kappus, 2004) showed that overall, it may be just as successful for a single screening question about alcohol use to be posed, because it fits in more naturally and comfortably in the flow of the helping interaction.

REGULATION AND CREDENTIALING IN ALCOHOLISM TREATMENT

Many treatment facilities are accredited by the Joint Commission, formerly the Joint Commission on Accreditation of Health Care Organizations. Most state governments accept Joint Commission accreditation as a condition for licensing treatment facilities and the receipt of Medicaid reimbursement. The commission's standards, methods, and mission may be viewed at http://www.jointcommission.org.

However, not all states use the commission to regulate and accredit treatment facilities. The other major national organization that accredits treatment facilities is the Commission on Accreditation of Rehabilitation Facilities. Its standards, methods, and mission may be viewed at http://www.carf.org.

Accredited facilities may be found by type and state. Alcoholism and addiction programs are grouped under behavioral health (BH), followed by specialty such as detoxification (Wells et al., 2007). State licensure standards vary considerably.

Alcohol and drug counseling, once separate fields and occupations, are by and large merged as of now. Two parallel system of credentialing exist:

- Credentials provided by the state affiliates of the International Certification and Reciprocity Consortium (ICRC/AODA), which has 73 member boards, 38 within the United States. The ICRC/AODA system, which began in the late 1970s, has a national exam, but state affiliates establish other requirements such as college degrees. They include educational requirements, largely borrowed from the social-work milieu, in 12 core areas of alcoholism counseling: screening, intake, orientation, assessment, referral, crisis intervention, treatment planning, client education, records and record keeping, and individual, group, and family treatment.

• Credentials provided by the National Certification Commission, an independent body affiliated with NAADAC, the Association for Addiction Professionals. The commission has three levels of accreditation.

States or ICRC/AODA affiliate boards may grant entry-level credentials to personnel such as New Jersey's recovery mentor associates and chemical-dependency associates or full addiction-counselor credentials to workers like New York State's credentialed alcohol and drug counselors. State licensure, a relative recent phenomenon, complicates this picture. State licensure usually requires completion of a college or university degree and/or a masters' degree in addictions or other behavioral-health or clinical disciplines. College and university curricula in addictions were first implemented starting at the end of the 1970s and grew over the next 20 years. Degree programs become preferred providers of alcoholism-counselor and addictions-counselor training, replacing a workshop model. A national network of addictions educators and programs in higher education, INCASE, was founded in 1990 (INCASE, 2011). INCASE promulgated standards for accreditation for higher-education curricula adopted by the new National Addiction Studies Accreditation Commission, which came into existence in December 2010.

The knowledge and skill base of addictions counselors is set forth in a document published by the Substance Abuse and Mental Health Services Administration (2006a). The full document, endorsed by all the professional bodies in the addictions field in 1998, may be viewed at http://www.nattc.org/resPubs/tap21/TAP21.pdf.

The median annual wage of substance-abuse and behavioral-disorder counselors in May 2008 was $37,030.

MODERN MEDICATIONS FOR ALCOHOL-USE DISORDERS

In the treatment of acute alcohol withdrawal, the use of benzodiazepine sedatives has been standard for decades. Most prominently, these include chlordiazepoxide (Librium), diazepam (Valium), and lorazepam (Ativan). These medications prevent seizures and reduce the physical and psychological effects of acute withdrawal syndromes. Such drugs are not used as a treatment to reduce drinking or reduce cravings; they are, themselves physically addictive although safe to use for the three to five days of alcohol detoxification.

These medications have been approved by the U.S. Food and Drug Administration for the treatment of alcohol-use disorders:

- Naltrexone, marketed as ReVia, Depade, and Vivitrol, is an opiate antagonist, blocking effects of drugs like heroin. It has been adapted for use with alcoholics, who lose the euphoric high but keep the more sluggish and sedative effects of alcohol. Research shows that naltrexone reduces craving for alcohol and that users have fewer relapses to heavy drinking and drink on fewer days than alcoholics who do not take the drug. It's a fairly expensive drug, at about five dollars per day. Some physicians are enthusiastic about Vivitrol, the injectable form of the drug (Enos, 2010), which the FDA approved for alcoholism treatment in 2006.
- Disulfuram, marketed as Antabuse, has been used for decades as an alcoholism treatment. Normally, the first breakdown product of alcohol, acetaldehyde, which is toxic, is in turn broken down by an enzyme to a nontoxic metabolite. Disulfuram acts to block that enzyme. Therefore, this toxic substance makes drinkers quite ill soon after drinking occurs, producing flushing, vomiting, headache, and chest pain. Users report that even using shaving lotion, which often includes a form of alcohol, triggers these responses.
- Acamprosate, marketed as Campral, affects two neurotransmitter systems involved in alcohol dependence. Studies have shown some promising effects on alcohol cravings.
- The class of antidepressants known as selective serotonin reuptake inhibitors (SSRIs) that includes fluoxetine (Prozac) has been tested for treatment of alcoholism. They show a moderate effect in reducing drinking, mainly among those who are abusing but not addicted to alcohol (De Sousa, 2010).
- Baclofen, a medication originally prescribed for symptoms of multiple sclerosis, has not yet been approved by the FDA for alcoholism treatment, but it has shown efficacy in reduction of cravings and of alcohol intake among alcohol-dependent people (Addolorato et al., 2002). Clinical trials by the National Institutes of Health are ongoing. For more information see http://clinicaltrials.gov/ct2/show/NCT00597701.

Some studies indicate that a combination of medications together with support groups and cognitive-behavioral therapy is the most effective use of these medications (Feeney, Connor, Young, Tucker, & McPherson, 2006). A study by Pettinati and colleagues (2010) found that for the treatment of alcoholism with co-occurring depression, a particularly difficult combination to treat, an SSRI antidepressant such as sertraline (Zoloft), a Prozac-like drug, together with an anticraving medication such as naltrexone, as well as cognitive-behavioral therapy, resulted in half of the patients remaining abstinent throughout the 90-day research period. Project COMBINE is sponsored by the National Association on Alcoholism and Alcohol Abuse to devise the best combinations (http://pubs.niaaa.nih.gov/publications/combine/index.htm).

There is no contradiction between taking medications and attending Alcoholics Anonymous. The AA pamphlet "AA Member—Medications and Other Drugs" clearly states that AA members should not play doctor and advise others on medication provided by medical practitioners or treatment programs.

CHAPTER 12

Alcohol Use among Women

Problem drinking has traditionally been thought of, and portrayed as, a male activity. This perception conceals the drinking of women, which they and their families often hide. It has prevented women from being the target of prevention and treatment services. In recent years, however, this condition has begun to change substantially.

PREVALENCE OF WOMEN'S DRINKING

In most regions of the world, men outdrink women, engage in more heavy drinking, exhibit more problem behaviors such as drunk driving, and are more likely to progress into alcohol abuse and dependence. However, in many countries since the 1990s, there has been some convergence in gender drinking patterns. In a majority of countries, a great deal of gender-segregated drinking has occurred (Wilsnack, Wilsnack, & Obot, 2005).

In the United States, women have lower rates of drinking than men, according to all standard measures, for the previous month surveyed:

- Any alcohol use—57.5 percent for men versus 45 percent for women.
- Binge drinking (five drinks within two hours at some point during the past two weeks)—30.8 percent for men versus 15.1 percent for women.
- Binge alcohol use (five drinks within two hours on five occasions during the past 30 days)—10.5 percent for men versus 3.3 percent for women.*
- Heavy alcohol use (more than two drinks per day)—22 percent for men versus 5.1 percent for women.*

Also, men are twice as likely as women to meet the criteria for alcohol dependence or abuse during a given year—10.5 percent for men versus

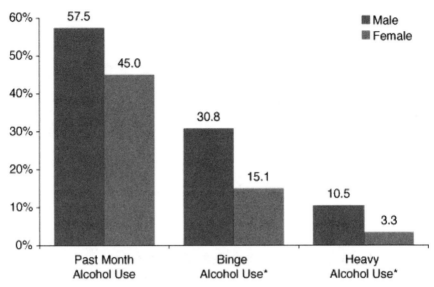

Figure 12.1 Percentages of past-month alcohol use among people ages 12 or older, by gender, 2004 and 2005 (National Survey on Drug Use and Health, 2007).

5.1 percent for women, and women who are divorced or separated and women between ages 18 and 25 are most likely to drink, and to drink heavily. (See figure 12.1.)

White women in the United States drink more than African American and Hispanic women. Middle-class white and African American women constitute the majority of moderate drinkers, with fewer abstainers or heavy drinkers. (On a graph, this is depicted with the familiar bell curve.) Among low-income African American women, more equal numbers of abstainers, moderate, and heavy drinkers produce a flatter graph. Church affiliation and being older correlates to abstention in African American women. More heavy drinking occurs among poorer white women than in the white middle class.

PHYSICAL ASPECTS OF WOMEN DRINKING

Female physical characteristics impact the degree and severity of intoxication and alcohol-related disease:

- Women have less body water than men of similar body weight, so they achieve higher concentrations of alcohol in the blood after drinking equivalent amounts of alcohol.
- Women appear to eliminate alcohol from the blood faster than men.

- Women develop alcohol-induced liver disease over a shorter period of time and after consuming less alcohol than do men.
- Women drinkers are more likely than men to develop alcoholic hepatitis and to die from cirrhosis.
- Although women have a much lower lifetime consumption of alcohol, heavy-drinking women show a rate of cardiomyopathy, or alcoholic heart muscle disease, similar to that of men.
- Even moderate to heavy drinking raises risks for breast cancer (National Institute on Alcohol Abuse and Alcoholism, 2004a; Su, Larison, Ghadialy, Johnson, & Rohde, 1997).

DRINKING AND DRIVING AMONG WOMEN

Although women are less likely than men to drive after drinking and to be involved in fatal alcohol-related crashes, women have a higher relative risk of driver fatality than men with similar blood-alcohol concentrations.

Women's lower rates of drinking and driving may be attributed to their lower tendency toward risk taking compared with men and because they are less likely to view drinking and driving as acceptable behavior. In one study, 17 percent of women, compared with 27 percent of men, agreed that it was acceptable for a person to drink one or two drinks before driving.

The proportion of female drivers involved in fatal crashes, however, is increasing. Between 1995 and 2007, the increase in the number of women ages 16 to 24 involved in fatal, alcohol-related crashes rose by 3.1 percent compared to an increase of 1.2 percent among young men (Tsai, Anderson, & Vaca, 2010). Yet the pace of female arrests for driving under the influence has greatly outpaced the actual rates of women driving drunk. Female DUI arrests skyrocketed by 28 percent between 1998 and 2007, while male DUI arrests declined 7.5 percent during that same period. These figures have been extrapolated in the media and on Web sites pertaining to substance-abuse prevention as meaning that there is an explosion in female drunk driving. High-profile cases like that of Diane Schuler, mentioned in the Preface, have seemed to give credence to this observation. Women, it is said, now take on more previously male-dominated occupational roles and associated stressors and are increasingly empowered to be risk takers like men (Join Together, 2009).

Some researchers believe that the lowering of the legally allowable blood alcohol concentration for drivers (from 0.10 of 1 percent to 0.08 of 1 percent) has netted more women than were previously arrested because they can more easily can reach that blood alcohol level with fewer drinks. In addition, instead of telling women, "Now drive home safely, dear," there is more stringent enforcement, and awareness, of women as drinkers and drivers (Schwartz, 2008; Schwartz & Rookey, 2006; Tsai et al., 2010).

RISK FACTORS FOR WOMEN

The myriad of risk factors cited previously in this volume apply to women as well as men. These include those of a genetic, developmental, and sociocultural nature.

As cited previously in chapter 13, two-fifths of people who started drinking before the age of 15 later acquired a diagnosis of alcohol-use disorder, and rates of alcohol dependence were 10 percent for people who started to drink after the age of 20 (Grant & Dawson, 1997). Women traditionally started to drink later than men, making them less at risk for developing alcohol-use disorders; however, that difference was eliminated by the end of the 20th century (Su et al., 1997).

Women who report having experienced sexual abuse, physical violence, or verbal aggression in childhood or adulthood are more likely to have alcohol-use disorders (Miller, Downs, & Testa, 1993; Wilsnack, Vogeltanz, Klassen, & Harris, 1997).

As mentioned previously, sex-segregated drinking, in which places for public drinking are reserved for men only, are the norm in many societies. This custom can have the effect of driving women into the closet, where their drinking is hardly noticed outside the home. Their alcohol symptoms can be rationalized or hidden as being caused by a cold or influenza, or by being out of sorts due to premenstrual syndrome. In Victorian and early-20th-century America, the all-male urban saloon was a widespread phenomenon, and groups such as the Women's Christian Temperance Union, under the leadership, most famously, of hatchet-wielding, six-foot-tall Carry Nation (1846–1911), campaigned vigorously against them (Lender & Martin, 1987; Pegram, 1998). The Prohibition era (1920–1933) created opportunities for men and women to drink together in the speakeasy subculture and at parties. The new custom of dating sprung up during that era, and the speakeasy was a dating destination, as were movie theaters, where many patrons brought hip flasks. Women were also heavily involved in the manufacture and distribution of alcoholic beverages. Finally, the Women's Organization for National Prohibition Reform, one of the major catalysts in the repeal of the Prohibition Amendment, claimed 1.5 million members (Pegram, 1998). Social historians disagree on whether women's drinking increased during Prohibition (Lender & Martin, 1987).

Despite the advent of integrated venues for socializing, all-male bars continued as a matter of custom or law for decades. The tradition flourished so strongly that in 1970, New York City enacted a law mandating that women be allowed to enter male-only bars. McSorleys Ale-House, on East 7th Street, for example, permitted women only after unsuccessfully fighting the law in court, with patrons and owners bemoaning the loss of this male refuge.

WOMEN WITH ALCOHOL-USE DISORDERS

Women who meet the criteria for alcohol-use disorders vary considerably by demographic characteristics. (See table 12.1.) Males outnumber females in all categories, but the figures differ by ethnicity and income.

Table 12.1 Percentages of Past-Year Alcohol Dependence or Abuse among People Ages 12 or Older, by Gender and Demographic Characteristics, 2004–2005

Demographic Characteristic	Male		Female	
	Percent	Standard Error	Percent	Standard Error
Age Group				
12–17	5.5	0.19	6.0	0.21
18–25	22.0	0.38	12.9	0.30
26–49	12.4	0.33	5.4	0.21
50 or Older	5.0	0.34	1.6	0.19
Race/Ethnicity				
White	10.6	0.22	5.6	0.15
Black or African American	9.7	0.62	3.5	0.27
American Indian or Alaska Native	19.5	3.83	13.7	2.52
Native Hawaiian or Other Pacific Islander	12.8	3.76	5.7	2.08
Asian	5.4	0.70	2.3	0.44
Two or More Races	9.9	1.28	7.7	1.27
Hispanic or Latino	12.1	0.59	3.8	0.27
Family Income				
Less Than $20,000	14.0	0.52	6.0	0.25
$20,000–$49,000	10.3	0.32	4.6	0.19
$50,000–$74,999	9.3	0.42	4.6	0.29
$75,000 or More	9.7	0.37	5.2	0.27

Source: Substance Abuse and Mental Health Services Administration (2006b).

As discussed previously, drinking patterns among African American women vary according to socioeconomic level. Other dimensions and factors in the incidence and prevalence of drinking and of alcohol-use disorders show stressors accompanying assimilation affect women's drinking and increase the risk of alcohol-use disorders. Gang membership is another factor in young women's development of alcohol-use disorders for many ethnic groups in lower socioeconomic brackets (Campbell, 1991).

Women are more likely to remain in relationships with alcoholic men than vice versa, and they may participate in drinking to keep the relationship afloat. Initiation of problem drinking may be tied to such a relationship. Alcoholic women in recovery are more prone to relapse when married, which contrasts with the recovery-sustaining role of marriage in men (Walitzer & Dearing, 2006).

Women develop drinking problems later in life than men, but they progress at a more rapid rate into alcohol dependence. This telescoping effect, which has been observed clinically and anecdotally for decades, is backed up by research (Johnson, Richter, Kleber, McClellan, & Carise, 2005; Randall et al., 1999). Important subgroups are adolescent young adults and widowed drinkers who descend rapidly into an alcohol-use disorder.

Woman alcoholics are more likely to have co-occurring psychiatric disorders, including depression, borderline personality disorder, and post-traumatic stress disorder, than men (National Survey on Drug Use and Health, 2004).

Women are less likely to be diagnosed with alcohol-use disorders or receive treatment for alcoholism. The stigma associated with alcoholism is most pronounced for women; women's drinking is more hidden within the home, both by status as mother or housewife, because of cultural taboos against their drinking, and because public drinking locations are male only in many cultures. More women are closet drinkers, but they have more support networks than men and are less likely than men to hit bottom. On the other hand, men engage in risk taking and drunken behaviors that get them arrested far more often than women. This problem behavior leads to treatment as an alternative to incarceration.

WOMEN IN RECOVERY TODAY

Traditional gender patterns in drinking have shifted in recent years with the public recovery advocacy movement. An important historic moment was the experience of then first lady Betty Ford. In 1978, the Ford family staged an intervention, and Ford entered the U.S. Naval Hospital for treatment of alcoholism and addiction to prescription pain medication following her struggle with breast cancer. Ford, already a prominent public advocate for women's health issues, went public with her story of recovery in the media and in her autobiographies *The Times of My Life* (1978) and *Betty: A Glad Awakening* (1987). In 1982, she founded the Betty Ford Center for Drug and Alcohol Rehabilitation, in Rancho Mirage, California, one of America's first prominent centers devoted solely to women's recovery, drawing celebrities including Elizabeth Taylor and Liza Minnelli. Ford received the Presidential Medal of Freedom (1991) and the Congressional Gold Medal (1999) for helping millions recognize their chemical-use problems and providing hope and inspiration for their recovery. One of the quotes ascribed to her in reference to her hidden alcoholism was, "My makeup wasn't smeared, I wasn't disheveled, I behaved politely, and I never finished off a bottle, so how could I be alcoholic?" Rates of women entering treatment have risen, and the stigma of having been a female alcoholic has lessened to some extent.

Among middle-class white women, there has been for some years a cocktail-mom subculture, although its existence is uneven among various ethnic and class groupings. According to a recent study, there is considerable influence on drinking that varies according to affiliation, with small clusters or networks that have norms of abstinence, moderation, or heavy drinking (Rosenquist, Murabito, Fowler, & Christakis, 2010). Changes in norms within these clusters have a great influence on drinking behavior. The drinking behavior of women, traditionally thought of as tied to the drinking of their mates, is now largely driven by their peers in the workplace or among clusters of mothers. The phenomenon of middle-class cocktail moms having a drink while socializing with other parents during a play date organized for their babies or toddlers had been relatively taboo. With the advent of blogging, however, the cocktail-mom subculture came out of the closet with blogs titled Mommy Wants Vodka and so forth. Even more recently, with horrific events such as the Diane Schuler incident, in which multiple alcohol-related fatalities occurred, women have questioned their own drinking habits and norms have changed in many peer clusters. Such changes in drinking norms spread into neighboring, connected clusters of women and thus affect wider networks (Rosenquist et al., 2010). We may add that these changes can also propagate within the blogosphere. Cocktail mom Stephanie Wilder-Taylor, author of *Sippy Cups Are Not for Chardonnay* (2006) and *Naptime Is the New Happy Hour* (2008), announced on her blog Make Mine a Double: Twins and Tequila, "I drink too much. I quit on Friday" (Hoffman, 2009).

In contrast to concerns about middle-class adult women, the media spectacle of alcohol abuse by young high-profile women such as Britney

Spears and Lindsay Lohan has resulted in a seemingly endless drama of public inebriation and personal deterioration interrupted by stays at celebrity rehab centers. Binge drinking among young women has been a concern in Europe, especially in the United Kingdom. In Scotland, in particular, there has been a media storm of coverage concerning youthful binge drinking and associated public inebriation and violence. In the United Kingdom, heavy drinking, and its physical consequences, among young women actually outstrips that of young men (Williamson, Sham, & Ball, 2003), even when the definition of *binge* is adjusted for gender (six drinks for women and eight for men, in the U.K. study).

CHAPTER 13

Alcohol Use among Adolescents

People have complained about adolescent behavior for over 2,000 years. Aristotle remarked that "youth are heated by Nature as drunken men by wine," and Socrates noted that adolescents are "inclined to contradict their teachers and tyrannize their parents." The heated nature of adolescence—the many risk factors that this transitional and contradictory period contain—contribute to a propensity to drink and be at risk for consequences such as automobile fatalities.

THE CREATION OF ADOLESCENCE

There is tremendous cultural variation in whether children move directly into adulthood or linger in a transitional adolescent phase. In some smaller, traditional societies, an entire birth cohort of youth may move into adulthood at one fell swoop in a mass ceremony. There has been dramatic cultural change in Western cultures: In England a thousand years ago, people were adult at 12, and in Germany 700 years ago, the legal code allowed 14-year-old males and 12-year-old females to marry without paternal consent (Bahr & Pendergast, 2007).

Adolescence as a recognized phase emerged at the start of the 20th century. Since then, adolescence has expanded into a ever-larger, protracted state: the age at which youths work, move out of their parents' homes, become financially independent, and marry, have been moved later and later, as seen in expressions such as "30 is the new 20" and terms like *adultolescence.*

A TIME OF CONFLICT

The paradox of adolescence as a category lies in its lack of definition. When one moves into adolescence, "a secure and established bio-social status is exchanged for a new status that is unsettled, marginal, conflictual, and uncertain of attainment...uncharted, ambiguous, and fraught with unknown implications" (Ausabel, 2002, p. 190); a process characterized by storm and stress, marked by conflicts with parents, mood disruptions, and risky behavior (Hall, 1904); identity crisis and role confusion (Erikson, 1968); a period when young people have a "confluence of unfaced dilemmas" (Levine, 1984, p. 141), a combination of isolation, boredom, drift, malaise, inability to conceive of a future for themselves, meaninglessness, difficulty in achieving or maintaining intimacy, a time when self-medication via alcohol/drugs, and a self-feeding alienation from family and community institutions are often in the cards.

Developmental psychologist Erik Erikson was the first to refer to the adolescent identity crisis, a period of role confusion (1975). Adolescence is a time when one is physically mature but not defined as an adult. There are conflicting motives concerning the approach to or avoidance of maturational tasks, intimacy, sexuality, romance, and independence. Conflicts create anxiety and put individuals at risk for depression and self-medication.

RITES OF PASSAGE

Every student who has had a cultural-anthropology course has heard of the rites of passage, or *rites de passage*. This is the universal human practice to ceremonially mark off the movement (passage) between social categories. Birth ceremonies such as baptism or ritual circumcision, marriage, and funerary rites are examples. Rituals that commemorate, celebrate, and mark off movement into adulthood are also near universal (Van Gennep, 1960). In many cultures, elders manage adolescent rites of passage, which involve imparting special knowledge and wisdom. In modern societies, these passage rites take place in a teen subculture and do not mark meaningful entry into responsible adulthood.

One of the major problems facing clinicians. prevention workers, and parents is precisely that substance abuse is one of the major American rites of passage.

Grob and Dobkin de Rios (1992) contrasted how adolescents managed consciousness alteration in rites of passage in three traditional societies with the dysfunctional use of drugs in American adolescence.

RISK AND FACTORS FOR ALCOHOL USE AND ABUSE

Adolescents and young adults are the population most mentioned as an at-risk age group for alcohol abuse. Two of the main reasons cited include the definition of alcohol use as a rite of passage and the nature of adolescence as a time of conflict, as described above. Other risk factors exist on many levels:

Broad societal risk factors exist. In the media, government, and the culture, alcohol use is portrayed as mature, sexy, sophisticated, leading to social acceptance, and facilitating social interaction. Alcohol and drug use is also defined as a tension reducer. Within ethnic, class, religious, and countercultural youth cultures, alcohol and drug use seen as rite of passage into adulthood. Gang, fraternity, and other cultures include heavy alcohol use. Risk factors in community networks and institutions (including school and church) include a lack of strong community-support systems, poor school resources, poor parent-school bonding, poor informal networks, and lack of powerful community-based religious institutions. Youth in communities favorable to drug use (such as those where men on street corners can be found drinking at 10 AM), where easy availability of alcohol is exemplified in concentrations of bars and liquor stores, are especially at risk. In addition, in communities with poor police-community relations, neighborhood disorganization, economic deprivation, and high rates of criminal activity, youth are susceptible.

The influences of immediate peers and kin and of family structure, support, conflict, and communication are also key. Factors in these areas include restrictive communication patterns within kin groups, intergenerational conflict and stress, alcohol-using peers and heavy alcohol use within family, parental psychopathology, family-member involvement with the criminal justice system; low expectations in the family for adolescents' academic careers, and parents' poor evaluation of adolescent peers.

In terms of individual psychosocial development, personality, and socialization, factors include favorable attitudes toward alcohol use, oppositionalism and rage toward family members, poor bonding to family members, experience of or witness to abuse, academic failure and low expectations of academic career, psychopathology and sociopathy, poor self-efficacy, boredom, meaninglessness, helplessness, and malaise.

Biological and genetic risk factors include nability to regulate modulate emotions and impulses, mood disorders, attention-deficit hyperactivity disorder, learning disabilities, and feeling more confident when intoxicated (Beman, 1995; Weinberg, 2001; Substance Abuse and Mental Health Services Administration, 1997).

Here is an example of how risk factors are interconnected and interactive:

In 1975, John has a genetic predisposition to be physically hyperactive, inattentive, and impulsive. He does not receive calm parenting from his mother and father, who are frustrated at their attempts to limit his behaviors. He is unpopular with his teachers, who find him to be a distraction in class, at best the "class clown." Rather than receive support for his ADHD, which has not yet been recognized as a diagnostic category, he is labeled as "bad," "lazy," "weird," labels which he internalizes, failing to develop a sense of his own potential and self-efficacy, further impacting his social and academic development. John also feels bored, isolated, and depressed. John was referred to counseling when he returned from lunch intoxicated.

Obviously, not all adolescents and young adults manifest all these risk factors, but it would seem impossible to avoid many of them as a person going through the maturation process. This is unparalleled in other age populations, and it leads to the epidemiological spike for these populations.

Although adolescents often maintain that their substance abuse is borne from a desire to have fun, feelings logs kept as homework in early-intervention treatment programs often reveal that there was a negative emotion that preceded use of alcohol or another psychoactive substance.

The level of risk varies significantly according to ethnicity. White non-Hispanic youth ages 12–17 reported the highest frequency of binge drinking, defined as having 5 drinks at a sitting. Among white youth, 9 percent reported binge drinking, compared to 6 percent of Hispanic youth and 3 percent of black non-Hispanic youth.

PROTECTIVE FACTORS AGAINST ALCOHOL ABUSE

According to studies funded by the National Institute of Drug Abuse, factors that protect against alcohol and other drug abuse among youth include:

- Family factors such as parental supervision and attachment by child to parent and vice versa.
- Educational factors such as higher reading and math percentiles, attachment to teachers and school, and positive parental values about college.
- Peer factors such as conventional values, positive attitudes toward law enforcement, and disapproval of daily drinking and public intoxication (Mathias, 1996; Smith, Lizotte, Thornberry, & Krohn, 1995).
- Personal factors such as language competence, high self-efficacy, and achievement orientation (Doll & Lyon, 1998).

The additive or synergistic effect of a number of specific protective factors forms a shield that holds steady for several years. Risk and protective factors are so important that they predict alcohol and drug abuse more than demographics such as ethnicity, gender, income, or age (Substance Abuse and Mental Health Services Administration, 1997).

BELIEFS ABOUT DRINKING

From table 13.1, one can see that from grades 8–12, the percentage of students who disapprove of daily drinking drops from 77 percent to 69 percent.

Table 13.1 Age and Ethnicity in Adolescent Disapproval of Drinking

	Disapproval of Daily Alcohol Drinking		
	26-16a. 8th Graders	26-16b. 10th Graders	26-16c. 12th Graders
Adolescents, 1998	Percent		
TOTAL	77	75	69
Race and Ethnicity			
American Indian or Alaska Native	DSU	DSU	DSU
Asian or Pacific Islander	DNC	DNC	DNC
Asian	DSU	DSU	DSU
Native Hawaiian and Other Pacific Islander	DNC	DNC	DNC
Black or African American	80	80	82
White	77	74	66
Hispanic or Latino	72	75	77
Gender			
Female	73	68	58
Male	82	81	80
Family Income Level			
Poor	DNC	DNC	DNC
Near poor	DNC	DNC	DNC
Middle/high income	DNC	DNC	DNC
Sexual Orientation	DNC	DNC	DNC

Data Source: Monitoring the Future Study, National Institute on Drug Abuse.

DNA = Data have not been analyzed. DNC = Data are not collected. DSU = Data are statistically unreliable.

Source: Substance Abuse and Mental Health Services Administration (2002–2007); National Survey on Drug Use and Health (2005).

But further down, one sees that African American and Hispanic students increasingly disapprove of daily drinking, whereas fewer of the majority whites cling to a temperance perspective. It is also significant to note that it is primarily female students who fall off the wagon in their beliefs during high school.

STATISTICS ABOUT ADOLESCENT ALCOHOL-USE DISORDERS

Alcohol use in adolescents predicts later misuse: Two-fifths of people who started drinking before 15 later acquired a diagnosis of alcohol-use disorder, and rates of alcohol dependence were 10 percent for persons who started to drink after 20 (Grant & Dawson, 1997).

Rates of alcohol-use disorders in adolescents don't show a great deal of fluctuation, while the ebb and flow in the use of marijuana, cocaine, and club drugs show a great deal of variation (see table 13.2).

TREATMENT FOR ADOLESCENT ALCOHOL-USE DISORDERS

If a teenager is drinking daily or getting drunk frequently, alcohol-abuse treatment may be indicated after appropriate screening and assessment. But treatment efforts borrowed from adult alcoholism-treatment models can be inappropriate and may be ineffective in stemming continued abuse after treatment is concluded. Rather, treatment should comprehensively target problems in all domains of functioning, including interpersonal adjustment, family functioning, academic problems, and learning disabilities and coexisting psychiatric problems (Liddle & Rowe, 2006; SAMHSA, 1998). Alternatives to alcohol use, sports and cultural activities, and involvement of the family are also important components.

Table 13.2 Percentages of Adolescents Meeting the Criteria for Substance Dependence or Abuse in the Past Year, 2002 to 2007

Substance	2002	2003	2004	2005	2006	2007
Alcohol	5.9%	5.9%	6.0%	5.5%	5.4%	5.4%
Illicit Drugs	5.6%	5.1%	5.3%	4.7%	4.6%	4.3%

Source: Substance Abuse and Mental Health Services Administration (2002–2007); National Survey on Drug Use and Health (2005).

Teens and Treatment

Being in treatment is associated with stigma, abnormality, punishment by adults, and perhaps more than in adolescence.

An adult will more likely have suffered much from drinking, and admit defeat in the long struggle with alcoholism, whereas a young person has not felt much of the harsh effects of his or her drinking and, in general, is more likely to have an omnipotent, invulnerable attitude.

An adolescent or college student will not want to enter any residential program that would result in missing a semester or year of school. For a teenager, that would be about the worst thing that could happen. Even an intensive outpatient program will take the young person away from his or her all-important social network.

There is a sense among many networks of adolescents that substance-abuse treatment is harsh and difficult. This perception is based on media coverage of alleged abuses at some tough-love and Outward Bound–type programs, as well as stories about old-style confrontational programs, which have, to a large extent, moderated their practices.

Some adolescents have difficulties with the deep spirituality of the Alcoholics Anonymous–based Twelve Step model utilized at many treatment programs. Other adolescents, however, can connect or reconnect to spiritual roots of their families and communities by participation in programs influenced by this model.

A program perceived as welcoming, nonstigmatizing, and empathetic, rather than punitive, will meet less resistance. Adolescents referred to treatment in the second decade of the 21st century are likely to meet counselors skilled in motivational interviewing (or a variation, motivational-enhancement therapy), discussed in our section on treatment (Miller & Rollnick, 1991; Center for Substance Abuse Treatment, 1999). This client-centered, user-friendly approach emphasizes working with clients at whatever stage of readiness to change they manifest. It views motivation as naturally ambivalent, dynamic, and fluctuating. Motivational-enhancement therapy is a good choice of a technique in working with adolescents for two reasons: First, it defuses the perception that the counselor-client relationship is an antagonistic one dominated by a punitive authority figure, which just inflames the normal rebelliousness of adolescence, which can be ramped up to intense resistance to treatment. Adolescents will appreciate the respect and empathy they have heretofore not experienced in their dealings with social institutions. Second, considering motivation as fluctuating, ambivalent, changing, and conflicted is more in synch with the adolescent spirit than with some set-in-their-ways adult.

CHAPTER 14

Alcohol Use among College Students

College drinking is a major concern of administrators and public health researchers. It has been seen a seemingly intractable social problem since the time of Thomas Jefferson almost 200 years ago, when he complained about rowdy, heavy drinking at the University of Virginia (Wechsler & Wuethrich, 2002). Programs to combat this phenomenon have come and gone, and there remains tremendous contentious debate on how to define and approach drinking at colleges and universities, which we outline in this section.

CENTURIES OF CAMPUS DRINKING

Heavy campus drinking waxed and waned during much of the 20th century. In a historical review, Room (1984, p. 541) noted that 1900–1910 was a decade of especially heavy drinking, quoting a 1903 campus survey to the effect that 90 percent of students were drinkers, that "35% drank heavily, and that 15% became drunkards." The period from 1910 to 1928 was comparatively dry, followed by a sharp spike in college drinking at the end of the 1920s, even during Prohibition. World War II lowered rates, which went up again at war's end as young returning soldiers went on campus. In recent decades, the rates of drinking and of heavy drinking on campus has held remarkably steady, contrasting to fluctuations in use of various drugs, and despite extensive prevention efforts (Wechsler & Nelson, 2008).

CONSEQUENCES OF HEAVY CAMPUS DRINKING

In 2005, 1,825 college students in the United States died from alcohol-related injuries, including vehicular crashes (Hingson, Zha, & Weitzman,

2009). That same year, 29 percent of U.S. college students admitted to have driven while drunk, up 3 percent from the previous year (Hingson et al., 2009). In 2002, over 500,000 full-time four-year college students were injured under the influence of alcohol and over 600,000 were hit or assaulted by another student who had been drinking (Hingson, Heeren, Zakocs, Kopstein, & Wechsler, 2002). At least one-half of sexual assaults on campus involve alcohol. In more than four-fifths of these alcohol-related campus sexual assaults, both the victim and the perpetrator had been drinking, 90 percent of the victims knew the perpetrator, and half happened on a date (Abbey, 2002).

A startlingly high percentage of students themselves report that during the current year, they experienced negative consequences due to their drinking (Core Institute, 2005). These consequences included that a student had

- gotten a hangover (62.5%).
- gotten nauseated or had vomited (54.1%).
- been hurt or injured (16.1%).
- experienced a memory loss (33.9%).
- missed a class (30.2%).
- performed poorly on a test or another project (22.1%).
- done something he or she later regretted (37.1%).
- been taken advantage of sexually (10.1%).
- gotten into an argument or fight (32.2%).
- had trouble with police or other authorities (13.9%).
- driven a car while under the influence (27.0%).
- been criticized by someone he or she knows (30.8%).
- thought he or she might have a problem (10.9%).

Heavy drinking adversely affects grades. One survey found a perfect inverse algebraic relationship between the number of alcoholic drinks and academic performance. Those who had 4 drinks or less during a week got A grades, those who took 6 drinks merited Bs, those who drank 8 drinks merited Cs, and those who imbibed 10 drinks got Ds (Presley et al., 1995).

WHICH STUDENTS DRINK AND DRINK HEAVILY?

The ages 18–21 represent a peak in drinking among all individuals, but college students drink more than nonstudents in the same age range. In fact, 45 percent of college students report a recent heavy-drinking episode (Hingson et al., 2009). Among college students, those of European descent (white) drink more than those of African American, Hispanic, and Asian descent (National Institute on Alcohol Abuse and Alcoholism, 1995b). Rates of drinking are low at historically black colleges and universities. In one study, 27 percent of African American students reported never having consumed an alcoholic beverage, compared to only 9 percent of white students. Of nonabstaining African American students, 20 percent hadn't had a drink in the past month, compared to only 10 percent of white students (O'Malley & Johnston, 2002; Siebert, Wilke, Delva, Smith, & Howell, 2003). Only 10–20 percent of African American students reported having had 5 drinks in a row during the past month (four for women), compared to 30–40 percent for Hispanics and 40–50 percent for whites.

College drinking is highest in the Northeast and North Central regions and lowest in the South and the West (Core Institute, 2005). Drinking and heavy drinking are lower at community colleges and nonresidential colleges. Where there is a significant presence of older students, minority students, and female students, rates of heavy drinking were moderated (Wechsler & Kuo, 2003). When those factors are combined, the results can be rates below the problem level. The lowest rate of alcohol consumption in New Jersey colleges and universities was that of Essex County College, a nonresidential community college with a median age of 25 and a predominantly African American and Hispanic enrollment, with negligible rates of heavy drinking. Drinking increases by college year attained. For males, the average number of drinks per week starts out at 7.7 for freshmen and reaches 9.2 by senior year. For females, the number of drinks starts out at 3.5 and reaches 4.2 by senior year (Core Institute, 2005; Stolberg, 1993).

In one study based on self-reported drinking (Knight et al., 2002), a startling 31 percent of college students met the diagnostic criteria as alcohol abusers, yet few sought treatment or were referred to treatment.

RISK FACTORS FOR HEAVY DRINKING
Beliefs about Drinking

Students believe that alcohol has many beneficial effects. Significantly more than half of students believe that alcohol breaks the ice, facilitates sexual opportunities, enhances social activity and peer connections in general, allows people to have more fun, and makes it easier to deal with stress (Core Institute, 2005). A majority believe that heavy drinking is a legitimate, normal, and expected rite of passage into college life (Crawford & Novak, 2006). However, factors cited in high rates of alcohol consumption and high-risk drinking patterns at colleges and universities include a carrying over of many or most of the adolescent risk factors cited above in the section on adolescence. Newly independent freshmen are feeling their oats but anxious about being away from home for the first time. They are greeted with the welcoming arms of entrenched drinking cultures on campus.

The role of alcohol marketing to students, availability of alcohol in bars and liquor stores near campus, and special promotions to students influences drinking (Kuo, Wechsler, Greenberg, & Lee, 2003). An example is that of Jägermeister, a reddish-brown German cordial having properties of root beer, licorice, and cough medicine, an unlikely candidate for campus popularity. The company that imports Jägermeister spent $6.5 million annually in the early 1990s (the only years for which data are available) to market the product in collegiate bars, with Jägermeister Parties, replete with promotional items, and Jagerettes, scantily clad young women who spray the beverage out of canisters into students' mouths (Beckwith, 1993). McCormick (1984) advised that "getting a freshman to choose a certain brand of beer may mean he will maintain his brand loyalty for the next 20 to 35 years. If he turns out to be a big beer drinker, the beer company has bought itself an annuity...today's youth market are tomorrow's high-volume drinkers" (pp. 10–11).

Fraternities and sororities were identified as hotbeds of inebriety almost from their inception in the first quarter of the 19th century (Horowitz, 1987). Today, Greeks still drink more than other students and engage in more heavy-drinking episodes. Fraternity-sponsored events also promote heavy drinking (Wechsler, Kuh, & Davenport, 1996). A study of one national fraternity, admittedly on the upper end of hard-drinking fraternities, reported that 97 percent of their members drank, with 67 percent frequently having 5 drinks in a row (Caudill et al., 2006). According to Park and colleagues (2009), heavy-drinking high school students self-select into fraternities and sororities and are in turn influenced by the heavy-drinking subculture found in them.

Pledging, hazing, and initiation have accounted for incidents in which a large amount of alcohol was consumed, resulting in alcohol poisoning and even deaths, which average about 25 in each of the last several decades (Nuwer, 1999). After one drinking death at Rutgers University, Chancellor Edward Bloustein angrily echoed 1950s anti-Communist rhetoric when he stated that "fraternities are a conscious conspiracy dedicated to the consumption of alcohol." Alcohol-prevention programming has been initiated at the highest levels of many national fraternities and sororities for some years now, including the North American Interfraternity Conference (North-American Interfraternity Council, 2009). These initiatives have sometimes been ignored or resisted by local chapters, and in fact fraternity drinking deaths have even occurred in fraternities promoting prevention initiatives (Nuwer, 1999). Mandatory alcohol training for fraternity and sorority leaders are important, as research indicates that Greek leaders set the tone regarding binge drinking (Cashin, Presley, & Meilman, 1998).

Collegiate drinking games and rituals are associated with alcohol poisoning. The twenty-first birthday is frequently an occasion where very heavy drinking occurs, and individuals interviewed a week before the event and after the event report that more drinking occurs than was planned (Brister, Wetherill, & Fromme, 2010). Drinking 21 shots at this event is also associated with alcohol poisoning and fatalities.

PREVENTION OF HARMFUL DRINKING AT COLLEGES AND UNIVERSITIES

Efforts to stem alcohol abuse on campuses have been made for decades. A comprehensive, institution-wide program endorsed by administration, faculty, and student leaders can send consistent messages that have the effect of changing campus culture (National Institute on Alcohol Abuse and Alcoholism, 2010).

Student-led, grass roots approaches show a great deal of value in alcohol-misuse prevention. These can include peer support groups, peer counseling, alcohol-information theater, peer education through curriculum infusion, and organizing a chapter of the national student network BACCHUS.

Other components of a campus alcohol-abuse-prevention program should include creating and enforcing policies concerning alcohol. This strategy can include instituting laws and regulations forbidding fake IDs, enforcing campus underage-drinking laws, working with local bars and liquor stores to enforce prohibition of sales to underage students, restriction of keg sales and beer sold in pitchers, restrictions on happy hours, restriction on billboards and other alcohol advertising, and regular meetings with local law enforcement to coordinate efforts. Knowledge and skill diffusion for staff and students is also essential. This approach can include bystander-intervention training, server training to screen for intoxication, screening and brief intervention for alcohol-use disorders, alcohol-refusal skills, recognizing the exaggerated misperception of peer norms and educating others about the issue, recognition of organizational denial of the problem on campus, education about alcohol and driving and alcohol and sexuality, and learning emotional coping skills that don't involve alcohol.

Students mistakenly exaggerate or misperceive how many of their class-mates use alcohol and other drugs and the amount they use, and demon-strating the accurate norms of drinking should reduce the rate of drinking (Perkins, 2003). Many prevention programs are predicated on that approach, and, in fact, became the basis for grant-funded prevention programs by various governmental entities. The National Social Norms Institute Web site (http://www.socialnorms.org/) lists a wide range of articles and stud-ies on this prevention approach. Many of Perkins's writings can be down-loaded from his academic Web site at Hobart and William Smith College (http://people.hws.edu/perkins/Publicat.htm). Dr. Berkowitz's writings, including an overview of the social-norms approach, are available at http://www.alanberkowitz.com. Michael Haines, a longtime leader of the social-norms movement, has a summary at http://www.higheredcenter.org/pubs/socnorms.html. However, Wechsler and Kuo (2000) claim that more stu-dents underestimate drinking on campus than overestimate it. Wechsler and colleagues also claim (2003) that there is no discernable reduction in drinking at campuses where social-norms campaigns take place. But many prevention workers believe that the norms strategy has a place in a comprehensive array of prevention activities.

CHAPTER 15

Alcohol Use among Older Adults

Until recent decades, the elderly had been almost automatically excluded from the discussion of alcohol abuse; dignified elders, it was long thought, surely do not belong in an account of drunken carousing and behavioral inappropriateness. Yet this approach is at variance with the statistical reality of alcohol consumption, and the health consequences thereof, among elderly populations. As the elderly population of the nation rises rapidly, it is in fact becoming an increasingly important public health issue.

OVERALL HEALTH CONCERNS

Heavy alcohol consumption has been associated with health consequences, including cirrhosis of the liver, motor-vehicle crashes, stroke, and other unintentional injuries (National Institute of Alcohol Abuse and Alcoholism, 1998a; Reynolds et al., 2003). However, light or moderate consumption has been associated with health benefits, including reduced rates of coronary heart disease and ischemic stroke (Breslow, Faden, & Smothers, 2003; Reynolds et al., 2003).

In one study of persons ages 60 or older (Eltner, 2010), one-third were found to be at risk for virtually all the problems associated with alcohol that have been described in this volume. Being male, white, and in the 60–64 age bracket, and having a lower level of educational attainment, accentuated the risk factors.

Although many medical and other problems are associated with both aging and alcohol misuse, the extent to which these two factors may interact to contribute to disease is unclear. Studies of the general population suggest that moderate alcohol consumption (up to 2 drinks per day for men and 1 drink per day for women) may confer some protection from heart disease. Although research on this issue is limited, evidence shows that moderate drinking also has a protective effect among those older than 65. Because of age-related body changes in both men and women, the National Institute of Alcohol Abuse and Alcoholism recommends that people older than 65 consume no more than 1 drink per day.

Alcohol-involved traffic crashes are an important cause of trauma and death in all age groups, but the elderly are the fastest-growing segment of the driving population. A person's crash risk per mile increases starting at 55 and exceeds that of a young, beginning driver by 80. In addition, older drivers tend to be more seriously injured than younger drivers in crashes of equivalent magnitude. Also, age may interact with alcoholism to increase driving risk. As older people's hepatic enzymes function less efficiently, they may achieve a higher blood-alcohol concentration at the same level of drinking. Coordination is also more easily impaired. For example, an elderly driver with alcoholism is more impaired than an elderly driver without alcoholism after consuming an equivalent dose of alcohol, and has a greater risk of a crash.

Falls are the most common injury for elderly adults. A great risk factor for falls and other accidents for the elderly is alcohol impairment. The incidence of hip fractures, other limb injuries, and craniofacial injury in the elderly increases with alcohol consumption. These increases can be explained by falls while intoxicated combined with a decrease in bone density in elderly persons, which is most pronounced in elderly people with alcoholism compared with elderly nonalcoholics (Johnston & McGovern, 2004; McLean et al., 2003).

Long-term alcohol consumption activates enzymes that break down toxic substances, including alcohol. Upon activation, these enzymes may also break down some common prescription medications. The average person older than 65 takes two to seven prescription medications daily. Alcohol-medication interactions are especially common among the elderly, increasing the risk of negative health effects and potentially influencing the effectiveness of the medications.

Alcohol exacerbates inactivity that increases the harm posed by chronic health conditions. Many elderly people complain of insomnia and may drink to sleep. However, alcohol interferes with normal sleep rhythms, and the drinker will awake fatigued.

ALCOHOL, AGING, AND MENTAL HEALTH

Depressive disorders are more common among the elderly than among younger people and tend to co-occur with alcohol misuse. Data from the National Longitudinal Alcohol Epidemiologic Survey demonstrate that, among people over 65, those with alcoholism are approximately three times more likely to exhibit a major depressive disorder than are those without alcoholism (Moos, Brennan, & Schutte, 1998). In one survey, 30 percent of 5,600 elderly patients with alcoholism were found to have concurrent psychiatric disorders. Among people older than 65, moderate and heavy drinkers are sixteen times more likely than nondrinkers to die of suicide, which is commonly associated with depressive disorders (National Institute of Alcohol Abuse and Alcoholism, 1998). The roots of late-middle-age and elder depression have to do with a range of factors.

Retirement can lead to the sense that one has lost the most important aspect of one's identity and one's most important role in life. This is mostly problematic with male retirees, who may feel worthless and obsolete. There is conflicting research on the effects of retirement on drinking. Though much prevention literature identifies retirement as a risk factor, Brennan and colleagues (2010) report a decline in drinking following retirement, because men no longer belong to groups that may drink on the job, at lunch, or after work. However, the approach to retirement and retirement itself may mean that the death of a dream that was never realized: Financial and occupational goals, and other life expectancies that had been hoped for, will never occur. In many U.S. ethnic groups, elders are not revered and valued as they are in many other cultures. Other losses in middle age and late middle age include grief and loss in the death of parents and other loved ones. Additional factors include the advent of the empty-nest syndrome as children move out and may relocate to distant locations, disappointment in the results of the aging process on the body, and a reduced sense of strength, vigor, and personal attractiveness and the loss of a positive body image. Physical pain, restriction of activities, and fatigue may accompany the aging process and chronic disease conditions for many older persons.

Having a strong support system is a major buffer against depression and emotional pain, but the social networks of the elderly are diminished by retirement and death.

In the isolation and inactivity that is often the plight of elders in solitary residence or in assisted-living facilities, ample opportunity exists to ruminate and relive losses, disappointments, slights, and painful memories.

Depression and alcohol misuse interact at many levels. Alcohol, of course, is a depressant. Alcohol will have an additive effect to medications that already have a depressant effect. And those who fear that their secret will be found out will increase their isolation from others.

EPIDEMIOLOGY OF ELDER ALCOHOL ABUSE

Although alcohol and other substance use is more common among younger adults (those ages 18–49) than among older adults (those ages 50 or over), the misuse of such substances among the elderly is quite high (Kohn, Corrigan, & Donaldson, 2000), increasing (Blow, 2000), and a major public health problem that leads to mortality, morbidity, and related health costs. It is difficult to find reliable statistics on today's elderly alcoholics. However, some research suggests that as much as 10–15 percent of the health problems in this population may be connected to alcohol and substance abuse (Moos, Brennan, Schutte, & Moos, 2004). Moderate amounts of alcohol tend to impair older adults more than younger drinkers because alcohol is metabolized and removed from the body differently in this population. Even moderate amounts of alcohol can cause measurable impairment for those over age 50. Alcohol use and abuse tends to be primarily a male problem among older adults (Thom, 2003). Social factors are a cause of vulnerability to alcohol use and abuse; however, it has been found that individuals who engage in excessive drinking may alter their social context. For example, older adults with money are more inclined to engage in social activities, have friends that condone drinking, and more likely to have problem drinking behavior (Moos & Holahan, 2010).

PROBLEMS IN IDENTIFYING AND CONFRONTING ALCOHOL USE AMONG THE ELDERLY

Alcohol abuse among older adults is something few in this population wish to talk about, and a problem for which even fewer seek treatment on their own. Too often, family members are ashamed of the problem and choose not to confront it head on. Health care providers tend not to ask older patients about alcohol use if it wasn't a problem in their lives in earlier years. These factors may explain why so many of the alcohol-related admissions to treatment among older adults are for first-time treatment.

Diagnosis of an alcohol-use disorder among the elderly is difficult because many symptoms, including aches and pains, insomnia, loss of sex drive, depression, anxiety, loss of memory, and other mental problems are often confused with normal signs of aging or the side effects of medications. Elderly patients, taking multiple medications, present an increased risk of medication-alcohol interactions, especially with tranquilizers and sedatives.

In late-onset alcohol-use disorders among elderly people, it may make less sense to treat drinking as a primary disorder and more sense to focus on the depression and isolation that are often the underlying factors (Smith, 2010).

CHAPTER 16

Alcohol Use among Ethnic Minorities

Discussion of any behavioral-health issue demands a grasp of group variation in belief and behavior. Competency in understanding cultural differences is a must in understanding alcohol use, and in constructing programs for prevention and treatment. This competency includes comprehension of differences in language, family structure and roles, beliefs and behavior regarding the supernatural, theories of the origin of behavioral and alcohol disorders, and patterns of communication.

DIVERSITY WITHIN ETHNIC GROUPS AND DRINKING

Ethnic categories in the United States are diverse in many ways, making any generalizations about their alcohol use a difficult business. Generalizing about, say, Hispanic drinking patterns is about as possible as generalizing about European drinking patterns. Aside from the shared language, the cultures of Spanish-speaking people are incredibly diverse, as are their drinking patterns. Rates of drinking by Mexican Americans are much higher than those of Puerto Ricans, which are again higher than those for Cubans (Nielsen, 2000). The same heterogeneity is seen in Asian Americans. It is often reported that they drink less than those of other ethnic minorities. Again, this finding obscures huge diversity among Asian ethnicities in America. More than 60 percent of Japanese Americans and more than 50 percent of Korean Americans reported alcohol use during the past month, whereas less than 30 percent of Americans of Chinese, Filipino, Indian, and Vietnamese heritage reported past-month drinking (Brown, Council, Penne, & Gfroerer, 2005). Up to one-quarter of Japanese Americans may be heavy drinkers, whereas the approximate rates for other Asian immigrant groups are lower; the figures are 20 percent for Filipino Americans, 15 percent for Korean Americans, and 10 percent for Chinese Americans (Kuramoto, 1995). Reasons for drinking also vary among Asian American ethnic groups. In one study of Asian American men in outpatient alcohol treatment (Park, Shibusawa, Yoon, & Son, 2010), almost half of Korean Americans reported drinking to relieve tension, as opposed to about one-quarter of Chinese Americans. Among Asian Americans, Korean Americans are referred to jokingly as the Oriental Irish (Kuramoto, 1995).

Socioeconomic status cross-cuts ethnicity. In the 19th century, people contrasted the "lace-curtain Irish" to the "shanty Irish." Drinking patterns of lower-income African Americans contrast greatly with those in the middle class.

The region of a country a person comes from and whether they are from an urban or rural area affect behavior once that person immigrates to the United States. New York City, for example, has both Mexican American residents who come from tough suburbs ringing Mexico City and those from rural areas who retain much of their Mayan cultural origins. Their drinking preferences and patterns also diverge.

Nations predominantly or entirely populated by immigrants have their own ethnic subdivisions: Cubans of Chinese or eastern European extraction, Vietnamese of Chinese extraction, and British of West Indian extraction alike live in the United States. Rates of heavy drinking in Protestant Northern Ireland have historically been a fraction of those in the Catholic Republic of Ireland, and these differences prevail among members of these subgroups who live in the United States.

Age and gender create important variations in drinking customs, patterns, and beliefs within ethnic groups. Among Puerto Ricans in New York City's South Bronx in the 1980s, a majority of older women believed that mental illness and alcoholism were rooted in supernatural causes, and they would refer an addicted family member to a spiritist, whereas younger and male individuals would more likely refer to conventional treatment (Myers, 1983). As opposed to a majority of Americans, who drink the most in young adulthood, heavy drinking among African Americans peaks in the 30s and 40s (Caetano & Herd, 1984).

British novelist Leslie Hartley opened his book *The Go-Between* (1953) with the epigram "The past is a foreign country—they do things differently there." Cultural changes within American society and within its constituent groups make any description of social behavior out of date in short order. A survey conducted among Latinos in the South Bronx revealed beliefs in, and willingness to refer to, folk-healing practices such as *espiritismo* and Santeria (a blend of Yoruba and Catholic beliefs and practices) for alcoholism and other behavioral and addictive disorders. Espiritismo traces behavioral problems to punishment by spirits for past deeds or deeds of ancestors, and to *corage*, or rages, that are also amenable to spiritual intervention (Myers, 1983). Yet few Puerto Rican college students questioned in 2009 had even heard of those hypotheses. Culture may also change very unevenly: Clothing styles and slang change at vastly different rates than, say, family structure and food mores. Many studies of Irish drinking, for example, are seriously outdated. Unfortunately, cultural-competency training in alcohol and substance abuse often relies on decades-old descriptions of ethnic behaviors.

Another complication is that stereotypes hide variation. Any description of cultural behavior identifies the most common or prevalent behaviors but can perpetuate a stereotype that does not fit many other members of an ethnic group. Probably the most famous and familiar example is the research on the use of personal space within cultures by Edward Hall (1966). Hall stated that northern Europeans and persons of northern European extraction stood further away from others during conversations than did southern Europeans, Arabs, Latin Americans, and those descended from those cultures, and even attempted to provide actual measurements. Nevertheless, it is obvious that many Norwegians, for example, will stand closer than many Italians or Egyptians. Quantification of behaviors or norms can conceal complexities. Denise Herd, perhaps the most prominent researcher on African American drinking, describes a profound ambivalence toward alcohol among American-born African Americans, even more than among other American ethnic groups, and even in the same community or family. There is a great temperance tradition in such environments, and a hard-drinking tradition as well. Or, in some communities where alcohol is integrated well into family and social life, liquor is negatively regarded (Herd, 1984).

ALCOHOL AND CULTURE AS A POLITICAL ISSUE

Ethnicity became an alcohol-use issue for the American public in the early era of temperance politics. More than 200 years ago, upwardly mobile African Americans who sought to improve their community, and who favored abolition of slavery, incorporated temperance as part of their crusades. In 1788, the Free African Society of Philadelphia did not admit drinkers. The founding planks of several African American religious denominations championed temperance as an integral tool for social reform and progress of the community. Fredrick Douglass considered temperance

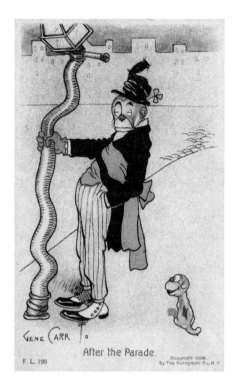

After the Parade.

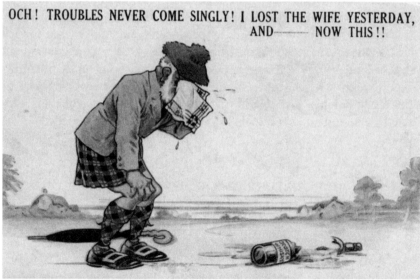

OCH! TROUBLES NEVER COME SINGLY! I LOST THE WIFE YESTERDAY, AND —— NOW THIS!!

Figures 16.1 and 16.2 Ethnic stereotyping of Irishmen (top) and Scotsmen (bottom) as drunks as seen in American postcards of 1910.

and the antislavery effort as inseparable, and regarded alcohol as a tool of the slaveholder both to keep slaves passive and to provide an outlet for their frustrations by dispensing alcohol on holidays and weekends and encouraged intemperance (Martin, 1986).

In the 19th century, nativist movements portrayed newly arrived ethnic groups, especially the Irish and the Germans, who began to immigrate to the United States in great numbers in 1840, not only as invaders but also as immoral drunkards. This kind of stereotypy continued up until the enactment of Prohibition in 1920, which Northern urban ethnic groups opposed and rural, Southern white Protestants championed (Lender & Martin, 1982).

ISSUES IN EPIDEMIOLOGY

Drinking differences within major categories such as African American, American Indian, Hispanic, and white are greater than the differences between them (Dawson, 2000). It is often reported that American Indians and Alaskan Natives have the highest rates of drinking, heavy drinking, and alcohol-use disorders, followed by Hispanics, African Americans, and finally Asian Americans. But these aggregate rates of drinking don't point to actual drinking pattern. For example, in a heavy-drinking episode, African Americans and Hispanics typically consume more drinks (8.4 and 8.1 drinks, respectively) than whites, who average 6.9 drinks per binge episode. Aggregate rates of drinking also do not necessarily correlate to medical and social consequences. For example, Hispanic males make up the group with the highest rate of death from cirrhosis of the liver, although they drink less, on average, than American Indians and Alaskan natives (Cremeens et al., 2009).

In 2001–2005, the Centers for Disease Control and Prevention estimated that 11.7 percent of all deaths among American Indians and Alaskan Natives were alcohol related, twice the percentage for all American groups. Primary causes were alcoholic liver disease and alcohol-related vehicle fatalities. Alcohol-attributed death rates were higher in American Indian groups throughout the Northern Plains states and lowest in the Southwest and Eastern United States (Centers for Disease Control and Prevention, 2008). Again, we must look beyond rates of drinking alone: The historically high rate of vehicle fatalities has also related to the prohibition of alcohol on reservations, which requires residents to drive long distances across rural areas to obtain alcohol. In addition, binge drinking is more prominent in reservation communities (May & Gossage, 2001).

THE PROCESS OF ASSIMILATION AND ACCULTURATION

Members of any given ethnic group are in transition from the culture of their nation of origin to the overall culture of the United States, or rather to the culture of the region of the United States in which they now reside. We use the term *assimilation* to refer to social integration and the word *acculturation* to taking on the lifestyle traits of the host culture. Members of ethnic groups range from those who have assimilated and acculturated hardly at all to those who have spent many generations in the United States, have successfully assimilated, and retain hardly any vestige of an ethnic culture of their own. Acculturating from a culture favoring abstention to that of the U.S. creates higher rates of use and lower rates of abstention. In one study, 75 percent of Mexican immigrant women in the United States abstained from alcohol, but only 38 percent of third-generation Mexican American women abstained. This rate is close to the 36 percent abstention rate for women in the general U.S. population (Gilbert, 1991).

Stresses associated with assimilation and acculturation are widely correlated with heavy drinking. These can include economic privation, isolation, intergenerational conflict, racism, and loss of important cultural symbols. The potential stress associated with migration and subsequent assimilation and acculturation can be buffered by strong ties to family and peer networks. Getting stuck while assimilating is also stressful and a risk factor for alcohol-use disorders. Two early portraits of how migration stress causes problem drinking were in studies of Mexican Americans in south Texas (Madsen, 1967) and Native Americans in Wisconsin and Michigan (Spindler & Spindler, 1971). In both, subgroups were identified that abandoned their traditional culture, but did not successfully assimilate with the mainstream culture, were discouraged and demoralized, and suffered from high rates of alcohol abuse. The Texas group was reviled by their countrymen as *agringados* ("gringo-fied," or Americanized). Native Americans who moved to Chicago and obtained stable employment had fewer heavy drinkers than those studied by Spindler (Garbarino, 1971). Groups in limbo, who are denied meaningful participation in the economy and society, feel a loss of face. Compounding this stressor is the common situation in which men have lost the status of breadwinner and are dependent on their wives' salaries or on systems of social welfare. Turning to strong drink compounds the marginalization.

Migratory and illegal immigrants have highly amplified stressors. Many illegal migratory workers from Mexico and Guatemala have had traumatic experiences in being smuggled into the country and constantly fear capture and jail or deportation, as well as isolation from their own families back home and isolation within the broader American society. Garcia and

Gondolf (2004) cite these factors as associated with their rates of heavy drinking, which stand out within the broader category of Hispanic or Latino. There are also high percentages of posttraumatic stress disorders among Mexican and Central American immigrants (Cervantes, Salgado de Snyder, & Padilla, 1989). Few of these individuals will seek out or are eligible for treatment for co-occurring alcohol-use disorders and PTSD, and they will often have folk interpretations of their problems, such as *susto*, which translates as "fright" but denotes soul loss due to trauma (Myers, 2002; Rubel, 1984). Many displaced people or people with trauma associated with immigration may turn to alcohol for succor. These include people with traditions of abstinence or moderation, including Cambodian refugee women (D'Avanzo, Frye, & Froman, 1994).

In the process of assimilating and acculturating, people and families may straddle two cultural worlds, with a bicultural, blended way of life. The New York Puerto Rican will say *rufo* for *roof* instead of *techo*, and *eleavador* instead of *ascensor*. A classic description of cultural blending in alcohol use was that of Howard Blane (1977), who compared immigrants and the children and the grandchildren of immigrants from Italy. Daily wine drinking plummeted fourfold across these generations and whiskey drinking picked up, but consumption of Italian wines and cordials stuck out as a trait not entirely given up. Other studies of Italian drinking (Simboli, 1984) show even further convergence with majority American norms.

The effects of immigration on alcohol use may vary greatly among ethnic subgroups Among Hispanic communities in a New England city studied by Andrew Gordon (1981), people from the Dominican Republic considered drunkenness as *indecente* and their drinking decreased after immigration; their norm of moderation was linked to their upward mobility and their attempt to be accepted in the local community. Guatemalan immigrants in the same city drank more after immigration, one-third engaged in frequent heavy drinking, and they romanticized drunkenness to the point that they would brag of a hangover when they had not drunk the night before. Puerto Ricans drank about the same after immigration, but some mixed alcohol with drugs, and family violence was also associated with drinking more frequently than among the other groups. Later studies of drinking among people from the Dominican Republic found a lifetime frequency of 22 percent for alcohol-use disorders, as opposed to 41 percent for Central Americans. For many, their transnational identity (many vote in Dominican Republic elections and have financial connections there) and their settlement in close-knit communities have slowed assimilation and buffered against acculturative stress. The theme of upward mobility continued: a majority of small groceries in New York City were owned by people from the Dominican Republic through the 1980s.

However, a minority have felt dishonored because of their inability to provide for their families and have detached from them and adopted the street life of alcoholics (Baez, 2005; Ricourt & Danta, 2003).

RECONNECTING AND RECOVERY

Reconnecting with traditional culture is a theme in recovery. This effort can be a facet of natural recovery without treatment as people mature out of alcohol abuse and reconnect with their religious roots. Ethnic pride or revitalization can also be an important component of a culturally competent treatment or prevention program. Among Native Americans, ethnic revitalization with a temperance theme has a long history. In 1799, the Seneca tribe, located in upper New York State, was living in a profound acculturative depression with high rates of alcoholism. Tribal member Handsome Lake had mystical visions that led to his own sobriety, and, under his leadership, contributed to the sobriety as well as the economic and cultural revitalization of the culture (Wallace, 1956, Wallce & Steen, 1970). Today, culturally competent programs such as the Red Road to Wellbriety, the Healing Forest, and the Talking Circle are pathways to sobriety for many Native Americans (White Bison, 2002; Coyhis, 2000). An epigram of the Red Road states,

> We may have misplaced our native Spirituality or sense of the sacred, but we can't say it's lost because we have ancestors within. Inside of us are grandmas and grandpas. When we start to come back to the culture they wake up, and we find that there are helpers both inside and outside. (White Bison, 2002, p. 34)

Efforts to integrate tribal traditions with evidence-based practices are also under way that target Native American populations entering alcoholism counseling (La Framboise, Trimble, & Mohatt, 1995). It is suggested that incorporating traditional religious elements into alcoholism treatment be broadened to include Thai Buddhism, Laotian Buddhism, Hmong shamanic treatment, Islam, the Eskimo Spirit Movement, and Latin American *curanderismo* and espiritismo. All these spiritual traditions share elements of suggestive symbolic rituals of healing and purification; confession, pledge, and sacrifice; reintegration into the community; and catharsis (Jilek, 1993).

PART II

Controversies

CHAPTER 17

Alcohol-Policy Perspectives

The term *policy* has many meanings, each depending on the context it is used, whether in national, social, health, or other milieus. Social policy may include principles or lines of argument that govern a course of action toward given ends by governmental and social institutions. Alcohol policies include:

- alcohol-related decisions made by legislators that are codified in the statutory language enacted in legislatures through laws.
- rules and regulations designed to implement legislation or to operate government and its various health-related programs.
- judicial decisions related to health (Longest, 1996; Block, 2004).

ALCOHOL POLICIES IN THE UNITED STATES

The Alcohol Policy Information System, funded by the National Institute on Alcohol Abuse and Alcoholism, provides detailed information about alcohol-related policies at state and federal levels. Such information covers 35 policy-related issues under the following topics:

- Underage drinking
- Blood-alcohol-concentration (BAC) limits
- Transportation
- Taxation
- Retail sales
- Alcohol-control systems
- Pregnancy and alcohol
- Health-care-services financing.

In the United States, federal, state, and local governments establish policies that govern the manufacture, sale, and use of alcohol and represent societal response to alcohol use and associated social problems. The legal basis for federal and state regulation of alcoholic beverages is derived from the U.S. Constitution. From 1919 until 1933, the 18th Amendment prohibited "the manufacture, sale, or transportation of intoxicating liquors" in the United States and its territories. At the end of 1933, Congress ratified the 21st Amendment, which repealed Prohibition and granted states broad powers to regulate alcoholic beverages.

Federal law can also influence state alcohol policies by means of financial incentives. For example, federal law requires that a portion of federal highway funding be withheld from any state that allows the purchase or consumption of alcoholic beverages by people under 21.

States vary in the amount of authority they allocate to local government to regulate alcoholic beverages. In many states, municipalities or other local government agencies create laws (often called ordinances) that regulate the sale and distribution of alcohol within their jurisdictions. In other states, alcohol control is retained at the state level with little or no regulation originating at local levels (Alcohol Policy Information System, 2010; Marin Institute 2011).

Policy Change

Table 17.1, from the National Institute on Alcohol Abuse and Alcoholism, shows policy changes from 1998 to 2009.

A specific example of alcohol policy is the U.S. surgeon general's report on preventing and reducing underage drinking (U.S. Surgeon General, 2007). Alcohol is the most widely used substance among America's youth—more so than tobacco and illicit drugs. (See the section on adolescents.) In response to the problem, the surgeon general's office released a statement of the following principles:

- Underage alcohol use is a phenomenon directly related to human development. Because of the nature of adolescence itself, alcohol poses a powerful attraction to adolescents, with unpredictable outcomes that can put any child at risk.
- Factors that protect adolescents from alcohol use as well as those that put them at risk change during the course of adolescence. Internal characteristics, developmental issues, and shifting factors in the adolescent's environment all play a role.
- Protecting adolescents from alcohol use requires a comprehensive, developmentally based approach that is initiated before puberty and

Table 17.1 Policy Changes at a Glance

Numbers in the table represent number of policy changes in each state per year

Policy Topic	1998	1999	2000	2001	2002	2003	2004	2005	2006	2007	2008	2009	Total
Underage Possession/ Consumption/ Internal Possession of Alcohol	1		1	2		1	2	2	4	1			14
Underage Purchase of Alcohol	2	2	2	1	2	2	2		1	1	1		16
Furnishing Alcohol to Minors	1						1	1	1				4
Minimum Ages for On-Premises Servers and Bartenders						1							1
Minimum Ages for Off-Premises Sellers											1		1
Use/Lose: Driving Privileges	1	2	1	2	1	3	1	3	2	4	2		22

(continued)

143

Table 17.1 *(Continued)*

Policy Topic	1998	1999	2000	2001	2002	2003	2004	2005	2006	2007	2008	2009	Total
Prohibitions Against Hosting Underage Drinking Parties			1		1		2	2	3	2	1		12
False Identification for Obtaining Alcohol		2	6	3	3	2	1	4	1	4	3		29
Blood-Alcohol-Concentration Limits: Adult Operators of Noncommercial Motor Vehicles		3	2	10	4	13	4	1					37
Blood-Alcohol-Concentration Limits: Youth (Underage Operators of Noncommercial Motor Vehicles)	5			1									6
Blood-Alcohol-Concentration Limits: Operators of Recreational Watercraft	1	4	2	8	2	9	1	2	2	1	2		34

Open Containers of Alcohol in Motor Vehicles	5	12	4	2			3		1	27
Vehicular Insurance: Losses Due to Intoxication										0
Alcohol-Beverages Taxes: Beer					5	1	3	3		12
Alcohol-Beverages Taxes: Wine					2	2	3	2		9
Alcohol-Beverages Taxes: Distilled Spirits					2		5	5		12
Alcohol-Beverages Taxes: Sparkling Wine										0
Alcohol-Beverages Taxes: Flavored Alcoholic Beverages								1		1

(continued)

Table 17.1 (*Continued*)

Policy Topic	1998	1999	2000	2001	2002	2003	2004	2005	2006	2007	2008	2009	Total
Keg Registration						7	2	4	1	4	2		20
Beverage-Service Training and Related Practices						1	5	4	3	1	1		15
Bans on Off-Premises Sunday Sales		1				3	2	1			1		8
Retail Distribution Systems for Beer	1				1	1		1		1	1		6
Wholesale Distribution Systems for Beer	1				1	1		1		1	1		6
Retail Distribution Systems for Wine	1		1			1	2	1			1		7
Wholesale Distribution Systems for Wine	1		1			1	1	1	1	1	1		8

Retail Distribution Systems for Spirits						1	1
Wholesale Distribution Systems for Spirits						1	1
Pregnancy and Alcohol: Warning Signs: Drinking During Pregnancy			2		1	1	4
Pregnancy and Alcohol: Limitations on Criminal Prosecution	1	1			1		3
Pregnancy and Alcohol: Civil Commitment	2			1	1	1	5
Pregnancy and Alcohol: Priority Treatment		1		1	1	1	3

(continued)

Table 17.1 (*Continued*)

Policy Topic	1998	1999	2000	2001	2002	2003	2004	2005	2006	2007	2008	2009	Total
Pregnancy and Alcohol: Legal Significance for Child Abuse/Child Neglect						3	2			1			6
Pregnancy and Alcohol: Reporting Requirements						2	3	2	2	2	2		13
Health-Insurance: Losses Due to Intoxication (UPPL)			1	1	3		1	1	2	3	3	1	16
Health-Insurance Parity for Alcohol-Related Treatment						3		1	1	1	1		7
	18	20	31	32	20	66	36	46	35	33	28	1	366

Source: National Institute on Alcohol Abuse and Alcoholism (2010a).

continues throughout adolescence with support from families, schools, colleges, communities, the health care system, and government.
- The prevention and reduction of underage drinking is the collective responsibility of the nation. Scaffolding the nation's youth is the responsibility of all people in all of the social systems in which adolescents operate: family, schools, communities, health care systems, religious institutions, criminal and juvenile justice systems, all levels of government, and society as a whole. Each social system has a potential impact on the adolescent, and the active involvement of all systems is necessary to fully maximize existing resources to prevent underage drinking and its related problems. When all the social systems work together toward the common goal of preventing and reducing underage drinking, they create a powerful synergy that is critical to realize the vision.
- Underage alcohol use is not inevitable, and parents and society are not helpless to prevent it (U.S. Surgeon General, 2007).

Based on these principles and the call for a healthy development of America's youth, the surgeon general proposed six goals for the nation that may be considered a policy position for the nation: The goals follow:

Goal 1: Foster changes in American society that facilitate healthy adolescent development and that help prevent and reduce underage drinking.

Goal 2: Engage parents and other caregivers, schools, communities, all levels of government, all social systems that interface with youth, and youth themselves in a coordinated national effort to prevent and reduce underage drinking and its consequences.

Goal 3: Promote an understanding of underage alcohol consumption in the context of human development and maturation that takes into account individual adolescent characteristics as well as environmental, ethnic, cultural, and gender differences.

Goal 4: Conduct additional research on adolescent alcohol use and its relationship to development.

Goal 5: Work to improve public health surveillance on underage drinking and on population based risk factors for this behavior.

Goal 6: Work to ensure that policies at all levels are consistent with the national goal of preventing and reducing underage alcohol consumption (U.S. Surgeon General, 2007).

The American Academy of Pediatrics statement "Alcohol Use by Youth and Adolescents: A Pediatric Concern" is another example of alcohol policy.

Alcohol use continues to be a major problem from preadolescence through young adulthood in the United States. Results of recent neuroscience research have substantiated the deleterious effects of alcohol on adolescent brain development and added even more evidence to support the call to prevent and reduce underage drinking. Pediatricians should be knowledgeable about substance abuse to be able to recognize risk factors for alcohol and other substance abuse among youth, screen for use, provide appropriate brief interventions, and refer to treatment. The integration of alcohol-use-prevention programs in the community and our educational system from elementary school through college should be promoted by pediatricians and the health care community. Pediatricians should support promoting the media's responsibility to connect alcohol consumption with realistic consequences. Additional research into the prevention, screening and identification, brief intervention, and management and treatment of alcohol and other substance use by adolescents continues to be needed to improve evidence-based practices (American Academy of Pediatrics, 2010).

International and Global Policy Initiative

The World Health Organization (2010a) reports that there are 76 million people in the world with alcohol-use disorders, compared to about 15 million with drug disorders. Worldwide, alcohol causes 2.5 million deaths, 3.8 percent of the total mortality rate, and unintentional injuries alone account for about one-third of these deaths. Globally, alcohol consumption is rising, and all or most of that increase is found in developing countries with few methods of prevention, control, or treatment.

The WHO has prepared a draft global alcohol strategy (see http://apps. who.int/gb/ebwha/pdf_files/EB126/B126_R11-en.pdf) that introduces the challenges posed by harmful consumption of alcohol and its consequences. Among the policy-related challenges and opportunities are

- increasing global action and international cooperation in order to decrease the impact of alcohol and its increased availability.
- ensuring comprehensive action aiming to reduce the harmful use of alcohol, considering the diversity of related problems.
- according appropriate attention to the burden of harmful alcohol use among decision makers, especially in developing and low- and middle-income countries.
- balancing economic and public-health interests.
- focusing on equity in developing policies that aim to reduce existing social disparities around alcohol consumption (including providing

information on the relationship between alcohol and social and health inequity).

- strengthening information in order to fill prevailing knowledge gaps, in particular concerning the situation in low- and middle-income countries.

The WHO global strategy has the following main objectives:

- Raise global awareness on intersectoral problems resulting from the harmful consumption of alcohol (health, social, and economy).
- Increase governments' commitment to concretely address these problems.
- Emphasize the importance of alcohol determinants and their prevention.
- Maximize the support given to member states in their work on prevention of harmful use of alcohol.
- Strengthen stakeholders' cooperation.
- Improve dissemination, implementation, and monitoring of information.

GUIDING PRINCIPLES

Although a balance needs to be found between economic interest and public-health interests, it is the public-health interest that must generate interventions to reduce the harmful use of alcohol. This needs to happen in an equitable way, taking into account national particularities. Policies must encompass all alcoholic beverages and target drinkers and their peers—and simultaneously support nondrinkers.

NATIONAL POLICIES AND MEASURES

Through legal and/or nonlegal frameworks, monitoring these actions will ensure their most effective implementation. The coordination of relevant stakeholders will ensure the effectiveness of existing national policies. Health ministries play a crucial role in this effort.

The WHO recommended a group of 10 complementary target areas, based on scientific knowledge and evidence:

- Leadership, awareness and commitment.
- Health services' response: Beyond their role to provide prevention and treatment to drinkers and their entourage, health services must

raise awareness of the health, social, and economic consequences of drinking.

- Community action: Local actions are often the most appropriate; they can be supported by higher-scale actions.
- Drunk-driving policies and countermeasures: Drunk drivers represent a burden on society that increases the need for prevention and sanctions.
- Availability of alcohol: The level of alcohol-related problems results from its availability in general, and to vulnerable groups in particular. Several dimensions come into play, and they are targeted in the WHO recommendations.
- Marketing of alcoholic beverages: Marketing, especially to children and young people, is also responsible for the current Europe-wide problem. Industry uses increasingly innovative strategies to transmit messages that must be regulated.
- Pricing policies: The link between the price of a product and its consumption has been scientifically established. Increasing the price of alcohol is one of the most effective interventions to reduce harmful use.
- Reduce the negative consequences of drinking and intoxication by targeting its broader context.
- Reduce the public-health impact of illicit and informally produced alcohol: Illicit and informally produced alcohol is an increasing practice, particularly in low- and middle-income countries. Unsafe substances used in some beverages increase the dangers of consumption.
- Monitoring and surveillance: Every target area includes several policy options, the implementation of which will have to consider the specific national context (European Health Alliance, 2010).

The International Center for Alcohol Policies (2010), a nonprofit organization supported by major producers of beverage alcohol, expresses the following policy statement:

The vast majority of people who consume beverage alcohol do so responsibly and to enhance the quality of their lives. When consumed moderately and in a responsible manner by individuals with good health and dietary habits, who have no medical reason to refrain from drinking, beverage alcohol is associated with few risks of harm and has been reported to have some beneficial effects on health. Irresponsible consumption of beverage alcohol is associated with a variety of risks both to the individual and to the public in health, social, economic, and safety contexts. Irresponsible consumption refers to high levels of intake, either on single occasions or repeatedly, or to drinking in inappropriate circumstances or by those who should not be drinking at all. Alcohol policies need to be based on an objective understanding of available research about alcohol and should aim to create a reasonable balance of government regulation, industry self-regulation, and individual responsibility. (International Center for Alcohol Policies, 2011)

However, it notes that there are specific areas of concern relevant to alcohol policy that needs to be considered, including drinking and driving, drinking guidelines, drunkenness, extreme drinking, marketing, noncommercial alcohol, violence, and young people's drinking.

CHAPTER 18

Key Issues and Controversies

Alcohol is a pivotal issue around which major public controversy exists. Social movements, constitutional amendments and their repeal, and changes in drinking age are hotly debated, and major organizations battle for national policies to allow or disallow drinking, or drinking by youth of a certain age, or to establish the very vocabulary with which we try to grasp these issues.

WHAT SHOULD BE THE MINIMUM AGE AT WHICH YOUNG PEOPLE CAN LEGALLY DRINK?

Worldwide, there is tremendous variation in attempts to regulate drinking age, ranging from nations that set no minimum age up to the most stringent, requiring a person be 21 years old. The following list outlines the variations in legal drinking age throughout the world:

Eighteen nations have no minimum age.
Twelve nations have a minimum age of 16.
Eighty-five nations have a minimum age of 18.
Three nations have a minimum age of 19.
Three nations have a minimum age of 20.
Five nations have a minimum age of 21.

The United States belongs to a very small club of nations that sets the bar high, three years higher than the age at which people can vote, and consumption of alcohol is prohibited in 6 states. In 21 states, consumption is prohibited with exceptions, and in 18 others, consumption is simply not prohibited. In many of those 21 states with exceptions, consumption is allowed when a parent or family member is present, or in a private club or other venue, on private property, or for religious or medical purposes.

After Prohibition (1920–33), most states restricted youth access to alcohol by designating 21 as the minimum legal drinking age, or MLDA. This term refers to legal purchase and public consumption of alcohol. However, in the early 1970s, 29 states lowered the MLDA to 18, 19, or 20. Concurrently, the minimum age for other activities, such as voting age, was being lowered (Wechsler & Sands, 1980). Studies of the effects of the lowered MLDA have focused on the incidence of motor-vehicle crashes, a major cause of death for adolescents. In the 1970s, it was found that crashes, injuries, and fatalities increased significantly among teens when the MLDA was lowered (Cucchiaro et al., 1974; Douglass, Filkins, & Clark, 1974; Wagenaar, 1983, 1993; Whitehead, 1977; Whitehead et al., 1975; Williams, Rich, Zador, & Robertson, 1974).

With this research in hand, advocacy groups pressured states to restore the MLDA to 21, and thus 16 states increased their MLDAs between September 1976 and January 1983. Resistance from other states, and concern that minors would travel across state lines to purchase and consume alcohol, prompted the federal government in 1984 to enact the Uniform Drinking Age Act, which forced states to raise the MLDA to 21 by threatening to reduce federal transportation funds to those states that would not comply.

Subsequent studies have confirmed that when the MLDA goes down, injury and death rates increase, and when it goes up, death and injury rates decline (Wagenaar, 1993). In addition, a higher MLDA results in fewer alcohol-related problems among youth, and the 21-year-old MLDA saves the lives of well over 1,000 youth each year (Jones, Pieper, & Robertson, 1992; National Highway Traffic Safety Administration, 1989; Wagenaar, 1993). The effects on drinking patterns from the elevated MLDA seem to persist into the early 20s (O'Malley & Wagenaar, 1991).

Mothers Against Drunk Driving, probably the largest and most influential policy and advocacy group in the drunk driving prevention field, founded The Support 21 Coalition, which is devoted to support for a continuing MLDA of 21 (Mothers Against Drunk Driving, 2011).

ARGUMENTS AGAINST THE LEGAL AGE OF 21

In the opinion of some people, the drinking age of 21 is a bizarre and sole exception to the definition of adulthood. An 18-year-old can fight and die in battle, marry and raise a family, and help elect a president but must wait another three years before having a beer.

Furthermore, some people believe that the drinking age of 21 pushes drinking into a dark corner where heavy drinking and alcohol abuse is more likely, away from regulation, role models, and healthy influence. In many if not most nations, youth are gradually introduced into drinking within a normal, responsible, family context. Although fewer youth may be drinking, when they do drink it is likely to be in a heavy-drinking context, putting themselves and the public at risk.

It is also argued that the drinking age of 21 makes youth into rebels, lawbreakers, criminals, and deviants. As the leaders of the movement Drink Responsibly point out, the situation for youth is analogous to the Prohibition era, but just for that age group: "It is easy to see the culture of speakeasies, rum runners, and bathtub gin mirrored in the keg parties, pre-gaming, and beer pong of today" (Choose Responsibility, 2011).

Making all drinking by 18-, 19-, and 20-year-olds a violation of the law means that prevention strategies such as responsible drinking and drinking alternatives can't be part of a federally funded program for high schools or colleges. Alcoholism expert Victor B. Stolberg wrote on an addictions blog,

> Back in 1984, when I was running an Alcohol Awareness Program at the University of Buffalo, I took a position at odds with many in the field. Essentially, I suggested that from a programming perspective the raising of the then 18 to 21 year purchase age limit would severely restrict the abilities of colleges and universities to regulate alcohol consumption on campuses. At that time, programs and services were dealing with ideas of "responsible drinking," teaching moderation, safety concerns, limiting availability of quantities, providing other alternatives, etc. These types of programming initiatives were much less viable with the raise to the 21 year limit. (Stolberg, 2010)

Some research does not bear out positive results for raising the drinking age:

- In a study of youthful drinking in Massachusetts after it raised the legal drinking age, self-reported alcohol consumption did not decline in comparison with New York.
- College students in states with a legal drinking age of 21 did not have much difference in alcohol abuse compared with states with lower drinking ages.
- Single-vehicle automobile fatalities were actually more frequent in states with higher age restrictions (Hanson, 1999).

The organization Choose Responsibility, http://www.chooseresponsibil
ity.org, headed by the president of Middlebury College, supports lowering
the drinking age to 18. The Amethyst Initiative, consisting of 135 college
presidents, is an offshoot of Choose Responsibility (http://www.amethyst
initiative.org). A list of arguments in favor of lowering the drinking age
can be found at http://www.chooseresponsibility.org/for_legal_age.

WHAT IS BINGE DRINKING?

For at least a century, a popular definition of "binge drinking" referred
to people who went on an extended period of heavy drinking, perhaps to
the point of stupor, and during which they basically dropped out of their
normal activities and obligations for several days. A 19th-century word
for a *binge* was *spree*, and another term, dating from the 20th century,
was *bender*. Wild binges were thought to be either a phenomenon found
in late-stage alcoholism or a type of periodic drinking described by
E. M. Jellinek as "epsilon" alcoholism. (Schuckit, Rimmer, Reich, &
Winokur, 1971). Binge drinking was also associated with holidays and
quasi-holidays such as collegiate spring breaks, but not to a single night of
drinking.

In 1992 and 1994, Henry Wechsler, a prominent alcohol researcher from
Harvard University who heads its College Alcohol Study, defined "binge
drinking" as a man having 5 or more drinks at a sitting or a woman having
4 drinks at a time if it has occurred over the past two weeks (Wechsler &
Isaac, 1992; Wechsler, Davenport, Dowdall, Moeykens, & Castillo, 1994),
the so-called 5/4 measure. This definition has been in use by the Centers
for Disease Control and Prevention (2011) and even has found its way into
standard texts on alcohol and alcohol abuse (Kinney, 2003), and Web sites
and pamphlets of countless prevention programs.

Access to the major articles published by the College Alcohol Study is
available at http://www.hsph.harvard.edu/cas.

Controversy has surrounded this definition since it was authored. Critics
have complained that the 5/4 measure has nothing to do with any standard
definitions of a binge and that the 5/4 measure is too low to qualify as a sign
of problem drinking. This number of drinks, they argue, might be sipped
over the course of an evening without the drinker getting drunk or engaging in problem behaviors. By the 5/4 standard, a woman who went out for
pizza and had two beers, and later went to a party and drank two glasses
of wine, would automatically be categorized as a binge drinker. While we
might encourage the woman to moderate her consumption, it would not
be helpful to brand her a binge drinker. Body mass is a crucial factor in

inebriation. A linebacker might absorb 5 drinks to small effect, whereas a short, slender man would be under the table by the time he finished his fifth drink. This disparity is ignored in adhering to the 5/4 measure.

The 5/4 measure makes common, normal, or near-normal drinking behavior into a social problem, defining 44 percent of college students, for example, as binge drinkers. It also has the unintended effect of validating heavy drinkers and alcohol abusers, because they are lumped into a category of almost half of the population. The man who is drunk throughout the entire weekend is thrown into the category with the woman, above, who had the beer and pizza.

For Wechsler's response to common criticisms of his approach, see http://www.sedqa.gov.mt/pdf/downloads/presentations_journalbinge drinking.pdf.

In 2004, the National Institute for Alcohol Abuse and Alcoholism approved a new definition of "binge drinking" that pulls back from a measure based on a number of drinks:

> A "binge" is a pattern of drinking alcohol that brings blood alcohol concentration (BAC) to 0.08 gram percent or above. For the typical adult, this pattern corresponds to consuming 5 or more drinks (male), or 4 or more drinks (female), in about 2 hours. Binge drinking is clearly dangerous for the drinker and for society. (National Institute on Alcohol Abuse and Alcoholism, 2004)

This is the blood-alcohol-content (BAC) equivalent of that for drunk driving—that is, just shy of 1/10 of 1 percent, or a 1/1,000 blood-alcohol level.

The National Institute on Alcohol Abuse and Alcoholism (2004) goes on to define a drink as a beverage that contains half an ounce of alcohol (e.g., 12 ounces of beer, 5 ounces of wine, or 1.5 ounce of distilled spirits). It defines risky drinking as reaching a peak BAC ranging from .05 to .08 and a bender as two or more days of sustained heavy drinking (National Institute on Alcohol Abuse and Alcoholism, 2004). In other words, a bender is now what a binge used to be. The term "harmful drinking" is an alternative approach, one that emphasizes the negative effects of excess consumption of alcohol.

SHOULD ALCOHOLICS BE FORCED INTO TREATMENT?

Most alcoholics are forced into treatment by some combination of pain, circumstances, and/or pressure from family, friends, or authorities. The vast majority of alcoholics coerced into entering treatment stem from court-ordered treatment of persons convicted of drunk driving (Cavaiola & Wuth, 2002; Dill & Wells-Parker, 2006). Systems by which drunk drivers enter and receive treatment vary tremendously from state to state (see http://pubs.niaaa.nih.gov/publications/arh291/41–48.htm). Another major group of alcoholics coerced into treatment are people identified as needing an employee-assistance program. Many people achieve sobriety after referral to such a program and are thankful that someone cared enough to give them an opportunity to recover.

Arguments in favor of mandated treatment for alcoholism include:

- The life-saving benefit of forcing into treatment alcoholics who kill somebody while driving drunk.
- Alcoholism is a mental illness that renders drinkers irrational and unable to help themselves, and we are doing them a favor by getting them into treatment.
- There are tremendous quantitative and qualitative savings to society in health, legal costs, costs for incarceration, insurance costs, and pain and suffering of alcoholics and their victims.

Objections include religious or pseudo-religious tenets of programs that they are forced to attend (Brodsky & Peele, 1991). The state, some claim, does not have the right to police our consciousness, and some go as far to believe, as it might be stated, "I can choose to be drunk, and no government should be able to stop me."

Some people would rather face legal sanctions than be forced to expose their secrets and emotions in a highly charged group-therapy setting. It is difficult to draw a line when a person should be coerced into treatment. This view is based on values of self-determination and personal liberty. Finally, there is bias in the attention some individuals receive, while others can continue to drink without sanctions.

ARE ALCOHOLICS IN DENIAL?

A core belief among those involved with alcoholism treatment and recovery is that alcoholics are in powerful denial about their dependence on alcohol and the consequences of their drinking. Related to the to the denial view are strategies of minimization (exemplified in such statements as "I really don't drink too much," "I'm not that sick," and "I drink less than Ed") and rationalization (demonstrated by comments like "I only drink because my mother-in-law nags me," "I'm under a lot of stress right now," and "I'll cut down later").

Denial is the main topic of much recovery literature. Denial-related slogans, including "Denial: It ain't just a river in Egypt" appears on a line of recovery products including T-shirts, bumper stickers, and mugs.

A more recent competing view is that problem drinkers of various stripes have a yearning for normalcy at some level, even if it is not apparent. They attempt to cut down or limit the damage that their heavy drinking is generating. They would like things to be otherwise. They have a bundle of motives both for and against their problem drinking; this ambivalence is normal, shifting, and ongoing. To reduce this set of aspirations, fears, avoidance, and bravado to an intractable system of denial, it is said, would be a big oversimplification, one that will not help the problem drinker make healthy choices.

Another recent view, associated with the motivational-interviewing model, is that much of what counselors see as denial, is, in fact, an artifact of the counseling setting, where clients are being hit over the head with labels and drawn into a confrontation-denial trap (Miller & Rollnick, 1991). It is true that alcoholism counseling has featured confrontation of denial and the insistence that clients admit they are addicts and are powerless before their addiction. This admission, in fact, is the first step of the Twelve Steps of Alcoholics Anonymous. Even in the addictions field, it has long been a humorous observation that disagreement is too easily chalked up to denial. A student of one of the authors reported that "I had a problem running the group today because some of the members are in denial about being powerless over their addiction" (P. L. Myers, personal communication from student to professor, May 2010). Clearly, the problem was that the group facilitator was engaging in an argument over respective interpretations of the nature of problem drinking.

Some counselors and addictions educators have gone so far as to call for retiring the concept of denial. Michael Taleff, past president of the International Coalition for Addiction Studies Education, declared, "Let's deny that denial is so basic to addiction theory. Let's let it die" (Taleff, 1994, p. 52). Needless to say, traditional addictions counselors have roundly denounced his declaration and other statements of this type. Other clinicians take a middle ground, not wishing to dispense with the concept but noting that it is not helpful to batter people who have problems with more labels and accusations. Instead of accusing them of denial, they suggest, simply record that the person is not motivated to change in a particular area.

People with alcohol problems tend to disavow many aspects of their problems. They disallow that they are drinking more and more, that they can't stay away from alcohol for an extended period of time, and that once they start drinking, they don't seem to have much control over how much they consume. They also deny that they are missing work or school as a consequence of drinking, that they are harming or annoying others, that they are spending a lot of money on alcohol, that their health is suffering, that they feel bad and guilty about their drinking, and that they are sneak-' ing and/or hiding alcohol.

The roots of denial are quite complex, more so than has been imagined in the alcoholism field. Acceptance of the label of *alcoholic* is feared because it may mean that the next step is entry into what seems to be a threatening institution or program. Many, if not a majority, of problem drinkers or alcoholics are forced or mandated into treatment, and their disavowal of problems is simply a normal rebellion against the loss of their freedoms (Taleff, 1994). Heavy users of alcohol may be immersed in a subculture that sees the use as normal or even positive; college fraternities, for example, have been singled out as such a group. In this regard, alcohol abuse can be seen as a cultural rather than a personal problem.

The problem drinker or alcoholic, as stated above, has a complex bundle of motives for and against heavy drinking. Also, there is unbearable inconsistency between what is and what should be. This state is so dissonant, confusing, and anxiety producing that alcoholics simply disavow this area of their life.

The term *alcoholic* or *drunk* has a terrible shame and stigma attached to it, and no one wants to buy into such a label. It implies that the drinker is worthless, a bum, a failure. Nowadays, there is more open identification about having an alcoholic past. Members of Congress and celebrities join with the organization Faces and Voices of Recovery to say, in effect, "Yes, I was an active alcoholic, and I'm proudly celebrating my status as a person in recovery."

If a person has truly lost control over his or her drinking and has suffered serious consequences, it is a very traumatic experience, and the person needs to defend himself or herself from that trauma by disavowing the problems (Bean, 1978).

Being found out as an alcoholic brings about fear of humiliation and exposure, and consequences such as job loss or loss of one's children; people are concerned that families and friends will reject them or think less of them if they admit they have a drinking problem, and they may consider it a weakness, a moral failure, or a sign of mental illness. People with problem drinking behaviors or alcoholism may fear to change from the devil they knew, or fear that the attempt to change will fail. This attitude often prompts a disavowal of the issue.

Alcoholic amnestic disorder, or impaired memory, results in periods of time when the drinker has no memory. In addition, people with advanced alcoholism may suffer neurological impairment. This condition does not constitute a state of deliberate denial but causes an inability to intellectually grapple with the situation.

Members of families and other social networks participate in minimizing or rationalizing drinking problems, doing so out of fear or guilt, or unfamiliarity with alcohol problems or because they seem to gain something out of a situation in which a family member is impaired. Members of institutions and organizations to which a problem drinker belongs have multiple reasons to avoid the issue: keeping up appearances, embarrassment and anxiety about confronting the issue, a buddy system that discourages ratting out colleagues, an organizational culture that defines heavy drinking as a normal time-out activity (Myers, 1990).

THE FATE OF ALCOHOL ABUSERS

Does alcoholism progress inevitably? Or can alcoholics and alcohol abusers get better on their own? A key concept in the alcoholism treatment and recovery communities is that alcohol abuse and alcoholism are inevitably progressing phenomena. The introductory section of the "Big Book," the basic text of Alcoholics Anonymous, states clearly that alcoholism is a relentlessly progressive illness (Alcoholics Anonymous, 1976), and most of the stories of alcoholic careers that comprise much of the book note that alcoholism leads to insanity, death, or prison. Famous alcoholism researcher E. M. Jellinek conducted a poll of members of Alcoholics Anonymous in the 1940s that indicated that this concept of disease progression became the basis of a scientific definition of alcoholic disease. Subsequent researchers have noted that at that time, the Alcoholics Anonymous fellowship was largely composed of so-called low-bottom alcoholics who had indeed ended up is terrible shape, seemingly incapable of stopping the deterioration and decline in their personal and medical conditions due to their drinking.

As described elsewhere in this volume, Jellinek described phases of alcoholism but later broke down alcoholism into various species, as he called them, of which severe and uncontrolled alcoholism was but one subtype—the mark of what he referred to as the Gamma alcoholic. Meanwhile, however, an admirer of Jellinek, Max Meir Glatt, diagrammed the downward slide of the poor Gamma alcoholic, and a possible return, climbing up the slope to recovery (Glatt, 1958). This U-shaped chart has been disseminated in one form or another throughout treatment facilities and textbooks as the model of what happens when one drinks too much, and it became part of the American disease concept of alcoholism. The National Council on Alcoholism, largely backed by members of Alcoholics Anonymous, convinced not only the treatment community but also the medical establishment of the veracity of this model. Marty Mann, one of the first female members of Alcoholics Anonymous, declared,

> Alcoholism is a disease which manifests itself chiefly by the uncontrollable drinking of the victim, who is known as an alcoholic. It is progressive, which, if left untreated, grows more virulent year by year, driving its victims further and further from the normal world, deeper and deeper into an abyss which has only two outlets: insanity or death. Alcoholism, therefore, is a progressive, and often fatal, disease...if it is not treated and arrested. (Mann, 1958, p. 3)

Alcoholics tend to have a variety of careers in drinking. They may have patches of heavy or abusive use from which they rebound, they may stabilize at a moderately abusive, heavy-drinking level and never suffer ill health effects, or they may quit drinking via any number of pathways to sobriety.

CAN ALCOHOLICS EVER GET BETTER ON THEIR OWN?

The prevailing view in the alcoholism treatment and recovery community is that without participation in a formal recovery program, alcoholics have little if any chance of changing for the better. They may struggle to remain sober for a short period of time, holding on for dear life (white-knuckle sobriety, as it is called in Alcoholics Anonymous), but they inevitably fall back without meaningful involvement in a recovery program. Champions of this view point to the "cunning, baffling, powerful" nature of alcoholic disease; this phrase from the AA basic text (Alcoholics Anonymous, 1976, pp. 58–59) is used very widely in the recovery community. Recovering alcoholics are told, "While you're here in this meeting, your disease is doing push-ups outside the door" (Myers & Salt, 2007, p. 11).

In addition, both Alcoholics Anonymous and formal treatment provide a conscious framework for preventing relapse. In Alcoholics Anonymous, it is awareness of so-called stinking thinking patterns that lead one to BUD, or build up to drink, that can be self-monitored and monitored by the Alcoholics Anonymous sponsor, and the admonition not to isolate and to continuously attend AA meetings for reinforcement of sober messages and immersion in the self-help milieu. In formal treatment, there is a great deal of emphasis on relapse-prevention strategies, including reduction of irrational thinking patterns such as so-called catastrophizing and awfulizing (Ellis et al., 1988) and coping strategies for stressful life situations. There is even a strategy for preventing a small slip from turning into a full-fledged relapse. Without such a framework, it is said, alcoholics are not prepared to survive in a long-term attempt at sobriety.

That illicit drug users mature out of use has been recognized for half a century (Winick, 1962); heroin users can't stand life on the street, and marijuana users are tired of the burnout feeling, and they decide to buckle down and compete in the workplace. But there is much less dramatic evidence of natural recovery from alcoholism, with the notable exception of college students, who may tone down the binge drinking after the freshman year (Misch, 2007). On the other hand, current alcoholism authors point out that one should not scoff at natural-recovery stories. After all, one of the favored modern approaches, the Transtheoretical Stages of Change (Prochaska & DiClemente, 1982), was based on a study of cigarette smokers who quit on their own. An addictions educator noted that in classroom discussions of recovery, almost every time a student got up to describe his or her recovery through a 12-step program and/or formal treatment, another person got up to describe how he or she quit via a personal spiritual experience or simply a hard, cold splash of reality such as a bout of hepatitis, jail, or homelessness. Natural recovery from alcoholism, while less documented than that from illicit drugs, seems to be more likely among those with fewer social problems generated by abuse, and more reliable community and family support systems (Bischof, Rumpf, Meyer, Hapke, & Ulrich, 2007).

CAN ALCOHOLICS LEARN TO DRINK MODERATELY, OR MUST THEY TOTALLY ABSTAIN?

The belief that alcoholics must never drink again was the unchallenged wisdom of the treatment and recovery community until 1962, when an article appeared in the prestigious *Quarterly Journal of Studies on Alcohol* (Davies, 1962).

The researcher followed 93 problem drinkers and found that seven of them were able to return to controlled drinking with stability for seven years. He concluded that while patients should be advised to aim at total abstinence, it is not correct that no alcoholic can transition to normal drinking behaviors. This study, and others that followed it, provoked tremendous acrimony in the alcoholism field that has only recently moderated.

Perspectives
Against Moderate/Controlled Drinking

Many people believe that alcoholics who try moderate drinking strategies are playing Russian roulette, and that their lives are truly at stake. Bell (1963, p. 322) noted, "For every alcohol addict who may succeed in reestablishing a pattern of controlled drinking, perhaps a dozen will kill themselves trying." Attempting controlled drinking strategies means a constant fight against reprogression of abuse, and conversion to and continued membership in robust, committed subcultures of abstinence such as Alcoholics Anonymous is a crucial aspect of recovery. The view of many people is that this fact is ignored by wishy-washy moderation strategies.

In Favor of Moderate/Controlled Drinking Strategies

Meanwhile, many people believe that blind opposition to controlled drinking strategies reflects dogma, not science, and the feeling by recovering alcoholics in the counseling field that their sobriety depends on abstinence; many people and many lives, it is believed, are lost by presenting the overwhelming and daunting goal of never drinking at all, ever again. By not opting into controlled drinking, some people say, we define every drink as a relapse, and trigger the abstinence-violation stricture that says, in effect, "One drink equals one drunk."

A controlled drinking option might be best for some, who might later opt for total abstinence. The Institute of Medicine estimates that there are four problem drinkers for every alcoholic (Institute of Medicine, 1990). Many people are of the opinion that offering a moderation or controlled drinking option to such people permits enables outreach to many more affected individuals. If that strategy fails, the logic goes, they can then be referred to abstinence programs. Our communities are best served, moderation proponents say, with a service continuum tied to problem severity. Controlled and/or moderate drinking studies are being undertaken in clinical settings utilizing cognitive-behavioral approaches. Researchers are claiming success for alcohol users who were not severely deteriorated or physically addicted (Rotgers, Kern, & Hoeltzel, 2002). One program that offers abstinence and moderation options is called DrinkChoice. A brief description appears at http://www.fullspectrumrecovery.com/control/articles/uploaded/drinkchoice.pdf.

Opponents of this view protest that alcoholics will self-select for the problem-drinker/controlled-drinking strategy, and that problem drinkers will seek to stretch the boundaries of moderation to return to their abuse regimen. Clearly, careful screening and assessment tools are needed to make this approach work.

A national mutual-aid organization, Moderation Management (http://www.moderation.org), has started to expand face-to-face meetings. Moderation Management had two setbacks around the end of the last century. In one, founder Audrey Kishline relapsed and caused a drunk-driving fatality. In the other incident, a member confessed to a murder in an online

Moderation Management chat group, but few members bothered to report it (Harmon, 1998). The Kishline accident was seized on as a general indictment of moderation strategies, although she had, in fact, quit Moderation Management two months earlier to return to Alcoholics Anonymous (Humphreys, 2003).

CHAPTER 19

Rates of Alcohol Consumption Worldwide

This chapter describes alcohol consumption by regions and by nations within regions, by adults (over 15 years in age), as compiled by the World Health Organization (2004). Space does not permit a separate breakdown by gender, age, and social class in most nations outside of the United States.

People in European nations drink more alcohol by far than those in any other geographic region or continent. Annual use there rose from 14 liters per adult in 1961 to 17 liters in the late 1970s, then showed a significant decline in the period 1983–1995 to about 10 liters and then stabilized until 2000, the last survey year. Within Europe, we find yearly adult per capita rates as follows:

- Czech Republic, 16.21 liters
- Ireland, 14.45 liters
- Moldova, 13.88 liters
- France, 13.54 liters
- Germany, 12.89 liters
- Croatia, 12.66 liters
- Austria, 12.58 liters
- Portugal, 12.49 liters
- Slovakia, 12.41 liters
- Lithuania, 12.32 liters
- Spain, 12.25 liters
- Denmark, 11.93 liters
- Hungary, 11.92 liters

- Switzerland, 11.53 liters
- Russia, 10.58 liters
- Finland, 10.42 liters
- United Kingdom, 10.39 liters (World Health Organization, 2004)

This list is almost identical to the world of top-drinking nations world-wide. The actual top nation is Luxembourg, but the statistic is discounted, as many of its drinkers do not reside there. also, trends for the United Kingdom, especially among youth, have changed upward in terms of alcohol consumed and heavy drinking engaged in since this report came out.

NORTH AND SOUTH AMERICA

The Americas are the second-ranking area in terms of alcohol consumption, averaging 6 liters in 1961, 8 in the 1970s, and 7 liters in 2000. The Americas, of course, constitutes quite a diverse array of nations and cultures (World Health Organization, 2004).

In drinking, the Americas were led by a cluster of heavy-drinking Caribbean nations—Bermuda (12.92 liters), Santa Lucia (10.45 liters), the Netherlands Antilles (9.94 liters), the Bahamas (9.21 liters), and Dominica (9.19 liters)—although not all Caribbean nations had such high rates.

Venezuela weighed in at 8.78 liters and the United States came in at 8.51 liters. Barbados, Brazil, Chile, Columbia, Costa Rica, Guyana, Panama, Paraguay, Suriname, and Uruguay were all in the range of 4.5–7 liters.

Guatemala had the lowest per capita rate, 1.64 liters in the Americas, contrasting with the large amount of drinking and alcohol-use disorders among immigrants to the United States; this factor is noted in the section about ethnic groups.

In the United States, the percentage of drinkers in 2010 was 67 percent. Since the late 1930s, when the Gallup Poll first surveyed on this topic, this figure has swung up and down from a low of 55 percent in 1960 to a high of 71 percent in 1976. Of the two-thirds of U.S. residents who drink, about 14 percent drink very little—1–11 drinks per year—which means that about half of Americans drink regularly.

Demographically, church attendance is most associated with abstention, and lack of church attendance with correlated with drinking. Almost half of weekly churchgoers abstain totally from drinking, but only 25 percent of those who never attend church are abstainers. Interestingly, the percentage of those who drink correlates to annual income, from a high of 81 percent among those who make more than $75,000, declining in every income category to a low of 46 percent among those who make less than $20,000.

Beverage preferences also vary demographically: Beer is the favorite among men, especially young men, while women preferring wine. Beer is most popular in the Midwest, and residents of the East and West Coast prefer wine (Newport, 2010).

AFRICA

The rate of alcohol consumption on the African continent hovered at about 4 liters per year for the past half-century overall. However, at the edges of this norm were nations with very low rates of consumption, such as Niger (.11 liters), Guinea (.14 liters), Mali (.49 liters), and Equatorial Guinea (.86 liters), as well as heavy drinking rates in South Africa (7.81 liters), Gabon (7.97 liters), Burundi (9.33 liters), Swaziland (9.51 liters), and Nigeria (10.04 liters) (World Health Organization, 2004). Interestingly, neighboring Ghana had a much lower yearly rate (1.54 liters) than the continent's leader. Some communities in South Africa's Western Cape Province have very high rates of fetal alcohol syndrome (Centers for Disease Control and Prevention, 2003) that reflects high alcohol intake among women. Also, the overall figures for the continent, as well as the data for many of the nations reporting extremely small intake of alcohol, do not take into consideration the large amount of home-brewed beers that figure so heavily in their cultures, as described in the next section.

WEST PACIFIC

Annual alcohol consumption in Western Pacific nations and territories has increased from 1.5 liters per capita to 4 liters over the past half century (World Health Organization, 2004). These countries and dependencies include the various Pacific Island groups, Indonesia, Korea, and South East Asian nations.

One of the leading drinking nations in the Pacific is Australia, storied as a heavy-drinking nation, with an annual per capita adult intake of 9.19 liters, but neighboring New Zealand comes in at 9.79. Both of these nations drink more heavily than the United States, but not quite at the level of the champion Europeans.

Southeast Asian nations went from virtually zero liters to almost 2 liters per capita, per year over the last half-century. Taken together with the data for the Western Pacific nations, we see a rise in a large number of developing, industrializing nations.

ASIAN NATIONS

If we peel off the major Asian nations from their geographical regions, we see adult per capita yearly rates as follows:

- Thailand, 8.47 liters
- South Korea, 7.71 liters
- Japan, 7.38 liters
- Laos, 6.72 liters
- North Korea, 5.68 liters
- China, 4.45 liters
- Vietnam, 1.35 liters
- India, .82 liters (World Health Organization, 2004)

It is not clear whether regimes with tightly control information (such as China, North Korea, and Vietnam) are communicating accurate rates to the bodies that have submitted them to our worldwide overview by the World Health Organization. Also, much unreported manufacture and consumption of homemade alcohol occurs; this consumption may amount to one-third of actual use, thereby contributes to an artificially low figure of reported consumption. Therefore, Indian adults may in fact consume 1.2 liters per year, which is still in the moderate range. However, India also has a substantial minority of Muslims, who do not drink.

MUSLIM NATIONS

At the very bottom of reported use are the Muslim nations, with negligible reported use. Iran, Kuwait, Libya, and Saudi Arabia report no use of alcohol. However, it is possible that their health-information reporting is colored by theocratic ideological constraints that preclude admission of any alcohol use. The other Muslim nations include Algeria, Bangladesh, Egypt, Mauritania, Pakistan, Saudi Arabia, Somalia, Syria, and Yemen in the Middle East and largely Islamic Indonesia in Southeast Asia.

UNRECORDED CONSUMPTION OF ALCOHOL

The rates of drinking cited in the above statistics do not take into account the licit home brewing of beer and wine and the illicit home distillation of spirits, nor the smuggling of alcohol. Home manufacture of liquor and spirits contributes to illness and death in that other, poisonous alcohols such as isopropyl alcohol and methanol, or wood alcohol, may precipitate into the mix, as mentioned in section I. Home manufacture of alcoholic beverages can add to the reported rates for alcohol consumption. Writers have chronicled homemade and bootlegged liquor in Russia for centuries. Therefore, Russia is probably even higher up on the alcohol list of nations within Europe than the rates quoted above would suggest. Another indicator of this unreported consumption is the large number of alcohol poisonings in Russia. Deaths from alcohol poisoning were over 40,000 in 2001, probably a combination of tainted bootleg spirits and intense bouts of binge drinking. Alcohol poisoning is a problem throughout the former Soviet and Eastern Bloc nations, where unrecorded consumption may be as high as one-third (Rehm, 2003; Rehm et al., 2009; Stickley et al., 2007).

CHAPTER 20

Culture and Alcohol Use

Culture is the way of life of a human group, a system of belief and behavior, values, norms, symbols, and customs. Culture influences the greater meaning of alcohol use as well as the definition and regulation of drinking behavior. Alcohol is woven throughout the fabric of society and culture, its ceremonies and sacred beliefs. The study of alcohol and culture can be an encyclopedic, lifelong avocation, and in fact is the focus of a study group within the American Anthropological Association.

INTEGRATION OF ALCOHOL THROUGHOUT SOCIETY AND CULTURE

Alcohol use is a major factor in many societies, although the behavior varies from society to society and between broad cultural regions. In the wine-producing southern European countries, for example, alcohol is considered an integral part of a meal and a variety of social and ritual occasions; people drink daily, and though it promotes social interaction, drunkenness is discouraged (Babor, 1992; Wylie, 1964). Drunkenness is relatively uncommon especially when one considers that these countries lead the world in wine consumption, and children are introduced to wine gradually as a natural process. In contrast, northern European cultures consume more distilled spirits, alcohol is consumed to achieve intoxication, and heavy drinking has been predominantly a male activity (Babor, 1992), although this pattern of use tends to be changing with rising levels of alcohol use among females. The inhabitants of the region comprising Germany, Austria, the German-speaking segment of Switzerland, and the Czech Republic and Slovakia consider beer their national drink, and beer is produced by thousands of small, local breweries in addition to larger concerns, and encourage local festivals such as

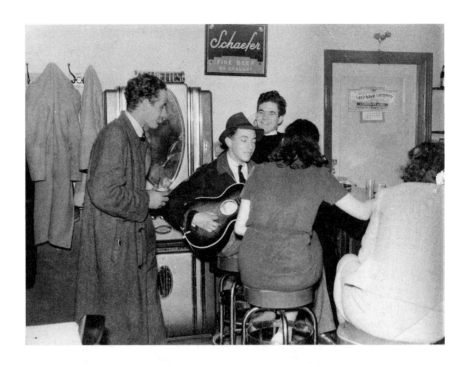

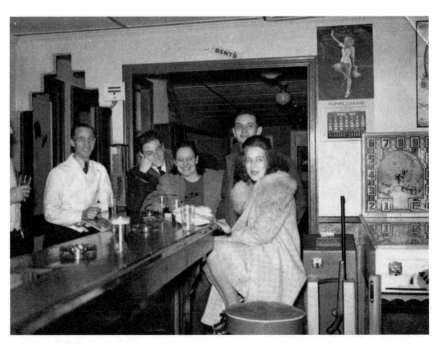

Figures 20.1 and 20.2 Informal photos taken in a genteel, family-oriented saloon in Plainfield, NJ, 1942.

those in springtime to introduce a new beer, as well as major events such as Oktoberfest (Bronisch & Wittchen, 1992).

In many societies, there is a specialized public place for drinking where information exchange, music, and recreation often occur. It is often an integral third place after work and home (Oldenburg, 1999); the traditional American saloon or inn, the Irish pub, the European café, and the African beer garden are a few examples. The classic study of the small Provençal village of Rousillon, in the south of France, showed the café as an institution that played the role of a public recreational center. It sold wine, tobacco, tax and postage stamps, and lottery tickets. It is a public living room for single adult males where everyone in town drops in for an aperitif (Wylie, 1964).

Drinking is a theme throughout the popular culture of many societies. Drinking songs are found worldwide; in American society alone, the joys and sorrows of drinking are celebrated in blues music, country-western tunes, and rap songs (Chalfont & Beckley, 1977; Connors & Alpher, 1989; Primack et al., 2007).

In Africa, beer drinking is pervasive and a central part of social events among the Itseo people of western Kenya, among whom there is a highly developed vocabulary pertaining to beer use and beer paraphernalia. Long-lasting relationships between people involve beer sharing with neighbors, who are defined as "people with whom one shares beer." Beer parties are organized where people form work groups that will work hard and accomplish a lot in a short period of time (Karp, 1980). The Kofyar people of northern Nigeria, meanwhile, "make drink, talk, and think about beer." Beer drinking is pervasive throughout social occasions, relationships, and significant events. A bride-price, or dowry, can consist of beer, and labor or rent can be paid with beer. The only words for short periods of time in the Kofyar language are based on the brewing cycle (Netting, 1964).

Among French people, wine drinking and the wine culture are characteristics of what it is to be French (Demossier, 2005). In their songs, Irish and Scots commemorate their identity as drinkers, and it has been said that the Irish used to drink because of economic and cultural conditions, but now they are Irish *because* they drink. Journalist Harry MacIntire (2006) blames the Scottish self-image of drinking as contributory to high rates of binge drinking, citing various literary sources that portray drunks as heroes and linking whiskey to liberty. The Scottish national poet, Robert Burns (1759–1796) wrote, "Freedom and whiskey gang thegither" ("Freedom and whiskey go together"), and consider this verse passage:

> Gie him strong drink until he wink…and liquour good to fire his blood….
> There let him bowse, and deep carouse / Wi' bumpers flowing o'er / Till he forgets his loves or debts / An' minds his griefs no more. (MacLean, 1993)

CEREMONIAL ALCOHOL USE

In a majority of traditional and small-scale societies, alcohol use is a ceremonial, ritualized activity. It serves to integrate the group and maintain communal solidarity. In many cultures, ranging from that of the Mongols to that of the Mexicans, the ritual importance of drinking is underscored by the fact that declining a drink is seen as disrespectful and unfriendly.

Certain ritual drinking practices, like buying rounds for the group and toasting, are widespread phenomena. The Chinese cultivate and value the skill of lengthy and loud toasting. In the Republic of Georgia, *tamada*, skilled toastmasters, have celebrity status; toasting at banquets and meals follows a formal pattern and involves everyone in the room; if the party is huge, assistant tamadas may be delegated to accommodate all participants. Even small, informal gatherings of men in cafés will elect a tamada, and their conversation will be structured as a series of toasts (Muehlfried, 2006).

In France, Israel, Mexico, Scotland, Spain, the United States, and many other countries, the most common toast is to wish health (Heath, 2000). Elaborate ritual handling of the glasses containing alcoholic beverages, including precisely how glasses are clinked, and with whom, are carefully followed in Japan and the Czech Republic.

Alcohol use is also an important aspect of rituals that call on the sacred and the supernatural. An early ethnographic expedition to the Yakut tribe in Siberia in the late 1800s recorded festivals involving fermented mare's milk, a recipe provided by the gods. There is the sacramental wine of the Catholic mass; the traditional Japanese house-building ceremony, in which food and sake are offered to the god of the carpenters and a ceremonial cup of sake is poured for all men present (Sargent, 1967); and the familial, sacramental significance of wine in traditional eastern European Jewish culture. Among the Itseo of Kenya, mentioned above, mortuary ceremonies are divided into five stages representing the progress of the deceased from the land of the living to the land of the dead, and each stage is associated with brewing and use of beer (Karp, 1980).

CULTURAL ATTITUDES TOWARD PROBLEM DRINKING

Culture defines problem behavior; cultures vary widely in what is considered an abusive level of drinking, in how badly one may act when intoxicated, and whether it is a problem that inebriates become aggressive in a bar or at home, or drive dangerously, or fail to arrive at work. Californians, for example, have defined drunken driving a problem of concern, while people of Mexico and Poland have focused on alcohol-related family disturbances and loss of productivity. Among many Czechs, however, failure to show up at work due to a hangover generates little guilt or criticism (Hall, 2005).

Culture defines what is serious or heavy use of alcohol. Consider this real exchange that occurred in the United States:

Counselor: Do you consider yourself a heavy drinker?
Client: No, I only drink beer.
Counselor: You were drunk when you came in the other day.
Client: No, we only had a few beers. (Myers & Salt, 2007, p. 311)

For this individual, as with many Americans, beer is considered a step above soda, and not an alcoholic beverage. A similar attitude is found among many Czechs as well (Hall, 2005). Furthermore, for many Americans, alcohol in general is not a drug, an attitude expressed in the statement "I never use drugs: I only drink."

Culture establishes values concerning alcohol. For example, many cultures consider heavy drinking, even self-destructive drinking, as manly (macho, to use the Spanish term), and romanticize this behavior: Picture, for example, Humphrey Bogart under a naked lightbulb trying to drown his sorrows in drink.

Culture defines the origin of problem drinking and alcoholism, whether it be moral failure or a supernatural influence. Traditional villagers in Mexico's highland state of Chiapas believe that when a person gets drunk, perhaps at the influence of demon trickery, the soul is paralyzed or leaves the body and is in great danger. Cures, it is widely believed, can be effected via the Catholic Church or by shamanistic healing (Eber, 2000). Culture defines drinking and heavy drinking occasions—that is, where one can drink, and how much. In the United States, there have been many informal workplace cultures of drinking, although these have fallen into relative disrepute over the past several decades. In Europe, studies show drinking separate from work environments; however, nonwork occasions are linked to heavy alcohol use and intoxification (Makela, 1986; Garvey, 2005).

The flip side of identifying drinking practices as problematical is romanticizing in the drinking practices of a nation. The Irish pub has become a cultural theme in many other nations. In Germany, especially Berlin, there is growing popularity for Irish-themed pubs, thought to import friendliness, relaxation, and conviviality, qualities associated in Germans' minds with the authentic venue (O'Carroll, 2006). Many American bars incorporate Irish themes in their name or decor as well, and there are reportedly Irish-themed bars in Siberia and Mongolia. Finally, Irish pubs are promoted within Ireland itself to promulgate tourism, and so this native cultural phenomenon has been to some extent turned into a commodity (McGovern, 2003). In addition, German-themed beer halls are found in the United States.

CULTURAL ROOTS OF ALCOHOL ABUSE

Many anthropologists have declared that in a majority of small-scale, traditional cultures, alcohol use is not problematic or socially disruptive, and the solitary drunkard is rare or nonexistent. When alcoholic beverages are defined as a food or a medicine or are integrated into the sacred and ceremonial life of a society, or both, problems are rare. Disruptive drinking almost never occurs in a sacred setting. In surveys of cultures around the world, problem drinking was associated with single-sex drinking, solitary drinking, the absence of group or community recreation leading to boredom, social disorganization, drinking with strangers, and drinking confined to nonreligious settings (Heath, 1975; Marshall, 1979).

Scholars in other fields criticize the idyllic view of traditional societies and have claimed that this romanticization leads anthropologists to deflate problem drinking (Room, 1984). In recent years, and with rapid social change transforming the majority of traditional cultures, anthropologists have revised their problem-free estimates of drinking in small-scale societies (Eber, 2000; Marshall, 1991).

The sudden introduction of alcohol into a society that has not had a chance to fully develop a comprehensive set of values and beliefs regarding its use is associated with alcoholism and problem drinking. Two examples are the so-called gin epidemic in London in the 1700s and the introduction of alcohol to Native Americans later in that century. Alcohol abuse is linked to rapid cultural change in general, and stress generated by migration— sometimes called acculturative stress—in particular, which may affect both individuals and entire communities where traditional culture is fragmented, undermined, diluted, or devalued, or where stress-buffering social networks are weak. Attempting, but failing, to step out and integrate with the dominant or host culture may be stressful in several respects, including in terms of economic deprivation and loss of status and self-esteem. To lose the role of breadwinner, or having to have one's children translate the dominant language, for example, communicates a loss of face.

HOW CULTURE SHAPES INTOXICATED BEHAVIOR

Pulque is a traditional Mexican beverage made from the fermented sap of the maguey, or agave, plant. According to one folktale, pulque was discovered by the opossum, who used his hands to dig into the maguey and extract the naturally fermenting juice that intoxicated him. Before the Spanish conquest, the Mexican Aztecs called pulque *centozonttotochtli*, or "400 rabbits," referring to the tremendous variety of effects that alcohol—in this case, pulque—has on the human organism (Marshall, 1983).

Intoxicated behavior and intoxicated roles are shaped by setting and expectations that are in turn largely defined by culture. MacAndrew and Edgerton (1969) proposed that drunken behavior—or, as they term it, "drunken comportment"—is socially learned and normatively regulated. Beliefs about alcohol and drunkenness are also socially learned. Alcohol use is often defined as a time-out, a "socially sanctioned time and place for doing many things that would be categorically inexcusable under normal circumstances" (p. 94)—for example, the office-Christmas-party effect. Many cultural traditions, from the bacchanalia of ancient Rome to the Carnival celebrations in New Orleans and in Central America and South America, feature a release of inhibitions, a time out from norms of social behavior, accompanied by heavy drinking. In highland Chiapas, this celebration occurs as what is translated as Crazy February, preceding Lent, when the natural order of things is turned upside down, men and women reverse dress, and anybody and anything can be mocked (Eber, 2005). The pharmacological disinhibition caused by beverage alcohol, the loosening of constraints on behavior, can mean many different things depending on set, setting, and expectation. Thomas Burns (1980) described young Bostonians who caroused from bar to bar, changing their demeanor from rowdy and raucous to quiet and deferential depending on whether they were in the downtown red-light district known as the Combat Zone or in Charlestown's mom-and-pop taverns.

Outright feigned intoxication, or pseudointoxicated state, are cited in a wide variety of cultures (Marshall, 1983), including the Rarotongans of the Cook Islands, the Truk of Micronesia, and the Aleuts, Chippewa, Naskapi, Salish, and Sioux and other Native American and Canadian tribes. In these cultures, people may become animated and festive before actually drinking or as a bottle is opened. Some stagger about after a single drink, or even after the first sip. Conversely, staggerers stop staggering when some event or task requires their attention and alcoholic aggression carefully misses forbidden targets. Brawlers cease brawling at a defined stage in life. Being drunk is invariably a public drama.

Anthropologists have examined the role of the drunk in several traditional societies. Being labeled as drunk provides an opportunity to send information without repercussion. At festive meals and other occasions in the village of Amilpas, in Oaxaca, Mexico, in the 1960s, an elaborate, polite front was always maintained. Animosities were denied and hidden behind this facade; someone was almost always there, to everyone's delight. to play the role of the truth-telling drunk. Drunks search out social gatherings, enter uninvited, and are very insistent on getting their information across (Dennis, 1979). Intoxicated Irish Tinkers or Travelers in Ireland in the mid-20th century engaged in bawdy sexual joking that would otherwise be considered scandalous. This behavior, and antagonistic attitudes, were excused with the remarks "The drink made him do it" or "It's the drink talking." Cross-cultural evidence reveals that some groups show little aggression when intoxicated and some are aggressive only in specific kinds of situations.

PART III

References
and Resources

Screening and Assessment Instruments

CAGE

C: Have you ever felt you should *c*ut down on your drinking?
A: Do you get *a*nnoyed when people talk about your drinking?
G: Do you feel *g*uilty about your drinking?
E: Have you ever had an *e*ye-opener, or a drink to get going after waking up?

Two or more yes responses to CAGE indicate a need for further screening and counseling (National Institute on Alcohol Abuse and Alcoholism, http://pubs.niaaa.nih.gov/publications/arh28-2/78-79.htm).

National Institute on Alcohol and Alcoholism Screening Questions for Heavy Drinking

1. Do you sometimes drink alcoholic beverages?
2. How many times in the past year have you had 5 or more drinks (if male) or 4 or more drinks (if female)?

A yes response to the first question and a response of one or more instances for the second question indicates a need to address alcohol consumption (National Institute on Alcohol Abuse and Alcoholism, http://www.niaaa.nih.gov/Publications/EducationTrainingMaterials/Documents/pocket.pdf).

Brief MAST (Michigan Alcohol Screening Test)

1. Do you feel you are a normal drinker?
2. Do friends or relatives think you are a normal drinker?

3. Have you ever attended a meeting of Alcoholics Anonymous (AA)?
4. Have you ever lost friends or girlfriends/boyfriends because of your drinking?
5. Have you ever gotten into trouble at work because of drinking?
6. Have you ever neglected your obligations, your family, or your work for two or more days in a row because you were drinking?
7. Have you ever had delirium tremens (DTs), severe shaking, after heavy drinking?
8. Have you ever gone to anyone for help about your drinking?
9. Have you ever been in a hospital because of your drinking?
10. Have you ever been arrested for drunk driving or driving after drinking?

Scoring:

< 3 points indicates nonalcoholic
4 points, suggestive of alcoholism
5 or more points indicates alcoholism

(Source: Pokorny A. D.; Miller B. A.; Kaplan H. B. (1972). The Brief MAST: A shortened version of the Michigan Alcoholism Screening Test. *American Journal of Psychiatry, 129*(3): 342–345.)

TWEAK

T—Tolerance: "How many drinks can you hold?"
W—Worried: "Have close friends or relatives worried or complained about your drinking in the past year?"
E—Eye-opener: "Do you sometimes take a drink in the morning when you first get up?"
A—Amnesia (stands for *blackouts*): "Has a friend or family member ever told you about things you said or did while you were drinking that you could not remember?"
K—Cut Down: "Do you sometimes feel the need to cut down on your drinking?"

Read more at: http://www.faqs.org/abstracts/Health/Alcohol-Screening-Questionnaires-in-Women-part-2.html#ixzz0ivUvbYQA

Alcohol-Use Disorders Identification Test (AUDIT)

Version 1: Short

1. How often do you have a drink containing alcohol?
2. How many drinks containing alcohol do you have on a typical day when you are drinking?
3. How often do you have 6 or more drinks on one occasion?
4. How often during the last year have you found that you were not able to stop drinking once you had started?
5. How often during the last year have you failed to do what was normally expected from you because of drinking?
6. How often during the last year have you needed a first drink in the morning to get yourself going after a heavy drinking session?
7. How often during the last year have you had a feeling of guilt or remorse after drinking?
8. How often during the last year have you been unable to remember what happened the night before because you had been drinking?
9. Have you or someone else been injured as a result of your drinking?
10. Has a relative, or friend, or doctor or other health worker been concerned about your drinking or suggested you cut down?

* The AUDIT is scored based on an answer range. Responses to questions 1–8 are scored as follows: Never = 0, less than monthly = 1, monthly = 2, weekly = 3, and daily or almost daily = 4. Responses to questions 9–10 are scored based on yes/no responses: No = 0, yes, but not in the past year = 2, and yes, during the past year = 4. A score of 8 or more is associated with risky drinking. Higher scores (13 or more for women and 15 or more for men) indicate the likelihood of alcohol dependence.

Version 2: Long

Please answer each question by checking one of the circles in the second column.

Q1	• Never • Monthly or less • 2–4 times per month • 2–3 times per week • 4+ times per week	How often do you have a drink containing alcohol?
Q2	• 1 or 2 • 3 or 4 • 5 or 6 • 7 to 9 • 10 or more	How many drinks containing alcohol do you have on a typical day when you are drinking?

(continued)

Alcohol-Use Disorders Identification Test (AUDIT) (*continued*)

Q3	• Never • Less than monthly • Monthly • Weekly • Daily or almost daily	How often do you have six or more drinks on one occasion?
Q4	• Never • Less than monthly • Monthly • Weekly • Daily or almost daily	How often during the last year have you found that you were not able to stop drinking once you had started?
Q5	• Never • Less than monthly • Monthly • Weekly • Daily or almost daily	How often in the last year have you failed to do what was normally expected of you because you were drinking?
Q6	• Never • Less than monthly • Monthly • Weekly • Daily or almost daily	How often during the last year have you needed a first drink in the morning to get yourself going after a heavy drinking session?
Q7	• Never • Less than monthly • Monthly • Weekly • Daily or almost daily	How often during the last year have you had a feeling of guilt or remorse about drinking?
Q8	• Never • Less than monthly • Monthly • Weekly • Daily or almost daily	How often during the last year have you been unable to remember what happened the night before because you had been drinking?
Q9	• No • Yes, but not in the last year • Yes, during the last year	Have you or someone else been injured as a result of your drinking?
Q10	• No • Yes, but not in the last year • Yes, during the last year	Has a relative, friend, doctor, or other health worker been concerned about your drinking or suggested that you cut down?

(continued)

Alcohol-Use Disorders Identification Test (AUDIT) (*continued*)

Your score on the AUDIT is _____.

A score of eight points or less is considered nonalcoholic, while nine points and above indicates alcoholism.

Your score of _____ does not indicate a problem with alcoholism.

A download of the AUDIT is available at http://www.niaaa.nih.gov/NR/rdonlyres/287137A9-62BF-4EDE-A752-4A351C57A0B8/0/Audit.pdf

Alcohol-Effects Questionnaire

This questionnaire consists of a series of statements that describe possible effects following alcohol use. We would like to find out about your present beliefs about alcohol. Please read each of the statements and respond according to your experiences with a heavy (5 drinks or more per occasion) amount of alcohol. If you believe alcohol sometimes or always has the stated effect on you, check Agree. If you believe alcohol never has the stated effect on you, check Disagree. Then, in the column to the far right, fill in the number that best corresponds to the strength of your belief, according to the following scale: 1 = Mildly believe 10 = Strongly believe. For example, if you strongly believe that alcohol makes you more intelligent, you would check Agree and enter a 10 in the far column. Please answer every question without skipping any. For a heavy (5 or more drinks per occasion) amount of alcohol

	Agree	Disagree	Strength of Belief
1. Drinking makes me feel flushed.			
2. Alcohol decreases muscular tension in my body.			
3. Drinking makes me feel less shy.			
4. Alcohol enables me to fall asleep much more easily.			
5. I feel powerful when I drink, as if I can really influence others to do what I want.			
6. I'm more clumsy after I drink.			
7. I'm more romantic when I drink.			
8. Drinking makes the future seem brighter to me.			
9. If I have had alcohol, it is easier for me to tell someone off.			

(*continued*)

	Agree	Disagree	Strength of Belief
Alcohol-Effects Questionnaire (*continued*)			

10. I can't act as quickly when I've been drinking.

11. Alcohol can act as an anesthetic for me; that is, it can deaden the pain.

12. I often feel sexier after I've been drinking.

13. Drinking makes me feel good.

14. Alcohol makes me careless about my actions.

15. Alcohol has a pleasant, cleansing, tingly taste to me.

16. Drinking increases my aggressiveness.

17. Alcohol seems like magic to me.

18. Alcohol makes it hard for me to concentrate.

19. After drinking, I'm a better lover.

20. When I'm drinking, it is easier to open up and express my feelings.

21. Drinking adds a certain warmth to social occasions for me.

22. If I'm feeling restricted in any way, drinking makes me feel better.

23. I can't think as quickly after I drink.

24. Having drinks is a nice way for me to celebrate special occasions.

25. Alcohol makes me worry less.

26. Drinking makes me inefficient.

27. Drinking is pleasurable because it's enjoyable for me to join in with other people who are enjoying themselves.

28. After drinking, I am more sexually responsive.

(continued)

Alcohol-Effects Questionnaire (*continued*)

	Agree	Disagree	Strength of Belief
29. I feel more coordinated after I drink.			
30. I'm more likely to say embarrassing things after drinking.			
31. I enjoy having sex more if I've had alcohol.			
32. I'm more likely to get into an argument if I've had alcohol.			
33. Alcohol makes me less concerned about doing things well.			
34. Alcohol helps me sleep better.			
35. Drinking gives me more confidence in myself.			
36. Alcohol makes me more irresponsible.			
37. After drinking, it is easier for me to pick a fight.			
38. Alcohol makes it easier for me to talk to people.			
39. If I have alcohol, it is easier for me to express my feelings.			
40. Alcohol makes me more interesting.			

Adapted from TIP 35 (Treatment Improvement Protocol 35), Enhancing Motivation for Change in Substance Abuse Treatment Appendix B – Screening and Assessment Instruments. Rockville, MD: U.S. Substance Abuse and Mental Health Administration, 1993.

Summary of American Society for Addiction Medicine Patient Placement Criteria

Dimension 1: Acute Intoxication and/or Withdrawal Potential—Risks associated with the patient's level of intoxication? Significant risk of severe withdrawal symptoms or seizures, based on the patient's previous withdrawal history, amount, frequency, and recency of discontinuation or significant reduction of alcohol intake? Are there current signs of withdrawal? Does the patient have the wherewithal to undergo ambulatory detoxification, if medically safe? Patient is rated 1, 2, 3, 4 on level of severity in withdrawal potential. 4, the most severe, would involve seizure, hallucination, possible liver failure.

(continued)

Summary of American Society for Addiction Medicine
Patient Placement Criteria (*continued*)

Dimension 2: Biomedical Conditions and Complications—Are there current physical illnesses, other than withdrawal, that need to be addressed because they are exacerbated by withdrawal, create risk, or may complicate treatment? Are there chronic conditions that affect treatment? Patient is rated from the mild 1 to the severe 4, which indicates incapacitation.

Dimension 3: Emotional, Behavioral or Cognitive Conditions and Complications—Current psychiatric illnesses or psychological, behavioral, emotional, or cognitive problems that need to be addressed, as they complicate treatment. Are such problems an expected part of the alcohol-use disorder, or do they seem to be a separate phenomenon? Even if connected to alcoholism, are they severe enough to warrant specific mental health treatment? Suicidal intent and level of threat. Ability to manage the activities of daily living. Again, patient is rated from 1 to 4, 4 requiring involuntary confinement due to life-threatening and dangerous behaviors.

Dimension 4: Readiness to Change—Is the patient actively resisting treatment? Does the patient feel coerced into treatment? How ready is the patient to change? If he or she is willing to accept treatment, how strongly does the patient disagree with others' perception that she or he has an alcohol-use disorder? Does the patient appear to be compliant only to avoid a negative consequence, or does he or she appear to be self-motivated way about his or her alcohol use? At what point is the patient in the stages of change: precontemplative, contemplative, planning to change, taking action to change?

Dimension 5: Relapse, Continued Use, or Continued Problem Potential—Is the patient in immediate danger of continued severe alcohol use? Does the patient have any recognition or understanding of, or skills in, coping with his or her alcohol-use disorder in order to prevent relapse, continued use, or continued problems such as suicidal behavior? How severe are the problems and further distress that may continue or reappear if the patient is not successfully engaged in treatment at this time? How aware is the patient of relapse triggers, ways to cope with cravings to use, and skills to control impulses to use or impulses to harm self or others? What is the patient's current level of craving to drink? Again, rated 1 to 4, 4 being the worst situation or most severe.

Dimension 6: Recovery Environment—Do any family members, significant others, living situations, or school or work situations pose a threat to the patient's safety or engagement in treatment? Does the patient have supportive friendships, financial resources, or educational or vocational resources that can increase the likelihood of successful treatment? Are there legal, vocational, social-service-agency, or criminal justice mandates that may enhance the patient's motivation for engagement in treatment? Are there transportation, child care, housing, or employment issues that need to be clarified and addressed? 1 would be a sober and supportive family, 4 might be a family or community consisting of other alcohol abusers.

(continued)

Summary of American Society for Addiction Medicine
Patient Placement Criteria (*continued*)

It is the combination of factors that has to be taken into consideration in deciding on what level of care the patient needs. In general, the patient would have to have 0 to 1 in all dimensions to qualify for outpatient treatment alone. Patients with some 2s and 3s might be destined for intensive day treatment; 3s and 4s would qualify them for residential rehabilitative care.

Alcohol Decisional Balance Scale

Client ID# _____ Date: ___/___/_____ Assessment Point: _____

THE FOLLOWING STATEMENTS MAY PLAY A PART IN MAKING A DECISION ABOUT USING ALCOHOL. WE WOULD LIKE TO KNOW HOW IMPORTANT EACH STATEMENT IS TO YOU AT THE PRESENT TIME IN RELATION TO MAKING A DECISION TO EACH STATEMENT ON THE FOLLOWING 5 POINTS:

1 = Not important at all, 2 = slightly important, 3 = moderately important, 4 = very important, 5 = extremely important

PLEASE READ EACH STATEMENT AND CIRCLE THE NUMBER ON THE RIGHT TO INDICATE HOW YOU RATE ITS LEVEL OF IMPORTANCE AS IT RELATES TO YOUR MAKING A DECISION ABOUT WHETHER TO DRINK AT THE PRESENT TIME.

How important is this to me?	Importance in making a decision about drinking:				
	Not At All	Slightly	Moderately	Very	Extremely
1. My drinking causes problems with others.	1	2	3	4	5
2. I like myself better when I am drinking.	1	2	3	4	5
3. Because I continue to drink, some people think I lack the character to quit.	1	2	3	4	5
4. Drinking helps me deal with problems.	1	2	3	4	5
5. Having to lie to others about my drinking bothers me.	1	2	3	4	5
6. Some people try to avoid me when I drink.	1	2	3	4	5

(*continued*)

Alcohol Decisional Balance Scale (*continued*)

How important is this to me?	Importance in making a decision about drinking:				
	Not At All	Slightly	Moderately	Very	Extremely
7. Drinking helps me to have fun and socialize.	1	2	3	4	5
8. Drinking interferes with my functioning at home or/and at work.	1	2	3	4	5
9. Drinking makes me more of a fun person.	1	2	3	4	5
10. Some people close to me are disappointed in me because of my drinking.	1	2	3	4	5
11. Drinking helps me to loosen up and express myself.	1	2	3	4	5
12. I seem to get myself into trouble when drinking.	1	2	3	4	5
13. I could accidentally hurt someone because of my drinking.	1	2	3	4	5
14. Not drinking at a social gathering would make me feel too different.	1	2	3	4	5
15. I am losing the trust and respect of my coworkers and/or spouse because of my drinking.	1	2	3	4	5
16. My drinking helps give me energy and keeps me going.	1	2	3	4	5
17. I am more sure of myself when I am drinking.	1	2	3	4	5
18. I am setting a bad example for others with my drinking.	1	2	3	4	5

(continued)

Alcohol Decisional Balance Scale (*continued*)

How important is this to me?	Importance in making a decision about drinking:				
	Not At All	Slightly	Moderately	Very	Extremely
19. Without alcohol, my life would be dull and boring.	1	2	3	4	5
20. People seem to like me better when I am drinking.	1	2	3	4	5

Scoring: Pros of drinking are items 2, 4, 7, 9, 11, 14, 16, 17, 19, 20. Cons of drinking are items 1, 3, 5, 6, 8, 10, 12, 13, 15, 18. To get the average number of pros endorsed, add up the total number of points from the items and divide by 10. Example: Pros of drinking = sum of items (2+4+7+9+11+14+16+17+19+20) divided by 10. To get the average number of cons endorsed, add up the total number of points from the items and divide by 10. Example: Cons of drinking = sum of items (1+3+5+6+8+10+12+13+15+18) divided by 10.

Adapted from TIP 35 (Treatment Improvement Protocol 35), Enhancing Motivation for Change in Substance Abuse Treatment Appendix B – Screening and Assessment Instruments. Rockville, MD: U.S. Substance Abuse and Mental Health Administration, 1993.

APPENDIX B

Alcohol Periodicals and Journals

Articles in the following journals are usually abstracted in CORK (Substance Abuse Information for Clinicians and Educators Database), Current Contents, DrugInfo, ETOH (Alcohol and Alcohol Problems Science Database), Excerpta Medica, Medline, and PsychInfo.

AA Grapevine (http://www.aagrapevine.org)

Addictive Behaviors: An International Journal (Elsevier Science Inc., http://www.elsevier.com)

Alcohol (Elsevier, http://www.elsevier.com)

Alcohol Alert (National Institute on Alcohol Abuse and Alcoholism, http://www.niaaa.nih.gov/publications/alalerts.htm)

Alcohol and Alcoholism: International Journal of the Medical Council on Alcoholism (Oxford University Press, http://www.oup.com)

Alcohol Research & Health (http://www.niaaa.nih.gov/publications/aharw.htm)

Alcoholism and Drug Abuse Weekly (Manisses Communications Group, http://www.manisses.com)

Alcoholism: Clinical and Experimental Research (Williams and Wilkins, http://www.alcoholism-cer.com)

Alcoholism Treatment Quarterly (Haworth Press, http://www.haworthpressinc.com)

American Journal of Drug and Alcohol Abuse (Marcel Dekker Inc., http://www.journals@dekker.com)

Drug and Alcohol Review (Taylor and Francis Inc., http://www.tandf.co.uk/journals/titles)

Employee Assistance Quarterly (Taylor and Francis)

Journal of Alcohol and Drug Education (JADE) (American Alcohol and Drug Information Foundation, http://www.unomaha.edu/~healthed/JADE.html)

Journal of Ethnicity in Substance Abuse (Taylor and Francis)

Journal of Social Work Practice in the Addictions (Taylor and Francis)

Journal of Studies on Alcohol (Rutgers Center of Alcohol Studies, http://www.rci.rutgers.edu/~cas2/journal)

Prevention Pipeline (National Clearinghouse for Alcohol and Drug Information, http://www.health.org)

Social History of Alcohol and Drugs (Alcohol and Temperance History Group, http://www.athg.org)

Substance Abuse (Taylor and Francis, Association for Medical Education and Research in Substance Abuse and International Coalition for Addiction Studies Education)

Bibliography of classic articles on alcoholism, http://www.projectcork.org/resource_materials/classicArticles.html

APPENDIX C

Additional Resources

Addiction Technology Transfer Centers (with links to individual regional centers; http://www.attcnetwork.org/index.asp)

Alcoholics Anonymous (http://www.aa.org)

As You Age (Substance Abuse and Mental Health Administration, http://asyouage.samhsa.gov)

BACCHUS Network (Boosting Alcohol Consciousness Concerning the Health of University Students, http://www.bacchusgamma.org)

Center for Substance Abuse Prevention (Substance Abuse and Mental Health Administration, http://csap.samhsa.gov)

Center for Substance Abuse Treatment (Substance Abuse and Mental Health Administration, http://csat.samhsa.gov)

College Drinking: Changing the Culture (National Institute on Alcohol Abuse and Alcoholism, http://www.collegedrinkingprevention.gov)

Do the Right Dose (Substance Abuse and Mental Health Administration, http://asyouage.samhsa.gov/dotherightdose)

Higher Education Center on Alcohol, Drug Abuse, and Violence Prevention (http://www.higheredcenter.org)

International Coalition for Addiction Studies Education (http://www.incase-edu.net)

Mothers Against Drunk Driving (http://www.madd.org)

NAADAC, the Association of Addictions Professionals (http://www.naadac.org)

National Black Alcohol and Addictions Council (http://www.nbacinc.org)

National Council on Alcoholism and Drug Dependence (http://www.ncadd.org)

National Institute on Alcohol Abuse and Alcoholism (www.niaaa.nih.gov)

National Latino Treatement Community Network (http://www.nlatinoaddiction.org/index.asp)

Rational Recovery (http://www.rational.org)

Reducing Alcohol Problems on Campus (Task Force of the National Advisory Council on Alcohol Abuse and Alcoholism, http://www.collegedrinkingprevention.gov/media/FINALHandbook.pdf)

Screening and Brief Intervention Kit for College and University Campuses (National Highway Traffic Safety Administration, http://www.friendsdrive sober.org/documents/SBI_College.pdf)

Students Against Destructive Decisions (formerly Students Against Driving Drunk, http://www.sadd.org)

Treatment Facility Locator (Substance Abuse and Mental Health Administration, http://www.findtreatment.samhsa.gov)

Unifying Principles of the 12 Steps of AA in the Wisdom Traditions (adaptations of Alcoholics Anonymous's Twelve Steps to various spiritual traditions, http://www.12wisdomsteps.com/index.html)

What's Your Poison? (Australian Broadcasting Company, http://www.abc.net.au/quantum/poison/alcohol/alcohol.htm)

White Bison Center for the Wellbriety Movement (http://www.whitebison.org)

Chronology

In this section, we present highlights in the history of the production, consumption, and regulation of alcohol from prehistoric China to 2011 in the United States. Depictions of intoxication and concerns about alcohol misuse figure in several ancient Middle Eastern cultures and persist throughout the history of the United Kingdom and the United States.

7000 B.C.   A fermented rice, honey, and fruit beverage in Jiahu China was produced (McGovern et al., 2004).

5000–4000 B.C. Viticulture (cultivation of vines for the making of wine) originated in the mountainous region between the Black Sea and the Caspian Sea, bordering Iran, Iraq, Syria, and Turkey. Origins of beer in Mesopotamia and Iran.

3000 B.C.   Sumerians maintained vineyards and also made alcohol from barley and dates.

2600 B.C.   The tomb of Methuen, a state official of Egypt, in Thebes, had paintings featuring a large vineyard. The hieroglyph for wine was a vine with bunches of grapes hanging down, supported by notched sticks on trellises. Alcohol was a reward for pyramid workers.

1700 B.C.   The law code of King Hammurabi (http://www.wsu.edu/~dee/MESO/CODE.HTM) included laws about the trade in wine, a low-status women's occupation, describing the consequences of breaking the laws, including these:

If a tavern-keeper (feminine) does not accept corn according to gross weight in payment of drink, but takes money, and the price of the drink is less than that of the corn, she shall be convicted and thrown into the water (Law # 108); If conspirators meet in the house of a tavern-keeper, and these conspirators are not captured and delivered to the court, the tavern-keeper shall be put to death (Law # 109).

1500 B.C.   Egyptian wine was fermented in open amphorae (ceramic vases), then sealed when fermentation was complete (Unwin, 1991, p. 69). Viticulture was established in mainland Greece.

1450 B.C.   The tomb of Antef of Thebes included the first known illustration of an intoxicated person, almost passed out near a wine-manufacturing facility. Other contemporaneous tomb paintings show two unconscious men being carried away by their servants from a banquet.

Old Testament   The Old Testament represented wine as a good and sacred thing, yet portrayed the evils of drunkenness:

Psalms 53:8–9: "You brought a vine out of Egypt, you drove out the nations and planted it; you cleared the ground for it, and it took root and filled the land."

Isaiah 5:7: "The vineyard of the Lord Almighty is the house of Israel."

Proverbs 20:1: "Wine is a mocker and beer a brawler; whoever is led astray by them is not wise."

Genesis 9:20–27 (New International Version): "...Noah's drunkenness and nakedness....Noah, a man of the soil, proceeded to plant a vineyard. When he drank some of its wine, he became drunk and lay uncovered inside his tent. Ham, the father of Canaan, saw his father's nakedness and told his two brothers outside. But Shem and Japheth took a garment and laid it across their shoulders; then they walked in backward and covered their father's nakedness. Their faces were turned the other way so that they would not see their father's nakedness."

Genesis 19:32–25, Lot's daughters get him drunk and commit incest: "Come, let us make our father drink wine, and we will lie with him, that we may preserve seed of our father....And they made their father drink wine that night: and the firstborn went in, and lay with her father; and he perceived not when she lay down, nor when she arose....And it came to pass on the morrow, that the firstborn said unto the younger, 'Behold, I lay yesternight with my father: let us make him drink wine this night also; and go thou in, and lie with him, that we may preserve seed of our father.' And they made their father drink wine that night also: and the younger arose, and lay with him; and he perceived not when she lay down, nor when she arose."

Habbakuk 2:15: "Woe unto him that giveth his neighbour drink, that puttest thy bottle to him, and makest him drunken also, that thou mayest look on their nakedness!"

Proverbs 23:29–35 (King James Version): "Look not thou upon the wine when it is red, when it giveth his colour in the cup, when it moveth itself aright. At the last it biteth like a serpent, and stingeth like an adder. Thine eyes shall behold strange women, and thine heart shall utter perverse things. Yea, thou shalt be as he that lieth down in the midst of the sea, or as he that lieth upon the top of a mast. They have stricken me, shalt thou say, and I was not sick; they have beaten me, and I felt it not: when shall I awake? I will seek it yet again."

Collapse of the Roman Empire. Viticulture was kept alive by monks. Wine was a sacrament representing the blood of Christ. In John II:1–11, Jesus turns water into wine at a wedding in Cana.

500 B.C. In Greece, Plato forbade use of alcohol to those under 18, permitted use in moderation to those under 40, and made no limits to those over 40. Policing of taverns was strict, and public drunkenness was punished.

400–500 B.C. Commentators in Athens such as Plato and Xenophon described a lively symposia discussion at which wine was drunk liberally. Greek wine was exported throughout the ancient world.

328 B.C. Alexander the Great killed his best friend Cleitus in a drunken rage at being contradicted for not following the counsel of his teacher Aristotle to practice moderation. Aristotle compared licentiousness to drunkenness, considering drunkenness as curable but licentiousness as permanent.

323 B.C. Alexander the Great died in Babylon following bouts of drunkenness.

300–200 B.C. In Rome, wine cultivation spread and became the basis of the Bacchanalia celebration in honor of Bacchus, the god of wine. Celebrations got out of control and had to be regulated. Cato the Elder (234–149 BC) called for moderate drinking and defended its medicinal value when infused with herbs. His book *De Agricultura* gives a comprehensive account of how to grow and process wine grapes.

A.D. 50 Roman philosopher Seneca the Younger, adviser to Nero, compared intoxication to addiction proper:

"The word *drunken* is used in two ways, in the one case of a man who is loaded with wine and has no control over himself; in the other, of a man who is accustomed to get drunk, and is a slave to the habit…there is a great difference between a man who is drunk and a drunkard."

65 Columella, a native of Roman Spain, wrote a 12-volume series on growing, processing, and marketing wine, *De Re Rustica*, and later *De Arborius*. The volumes describe the preparation of vineyards and the varieties of wine that can be produced by different strains of grape and methods of cultivation.

Pliny, in his *Naturalis Historiae*, listed 96 varieties of wine.

100	Winemaking was prevalent through the northern provinces of Rome, as were taverns, and there was considerable trade in Roman wines. The Roman elite supported its authority by distributing *mulsum*, or cheap wine, to the urban poor. Today, amphorae are still found along the coasts of the Mediterranean Sea.
200	Winemaking spread into the Danube Valley.
400	St. John Chrysostom, archbishop of Constantinople, decried the drunken habits of the citizens of Byzantium.
625	Muhammad ordered his followers to abstain from alcohol.
842–867	Byzantine Emperor Michael III was nicknamed the Drunkard.
900s	Anglo-Saxons maintained alehouses in Britain. In 997, Ethelred ("the Unready") decreed a fine when a fight in an alehouse led to someone's death and a smaller fine if no one is killed. The Anglo-Saxons drank *win* (wine), *meod* (mead), and *eolu* (ale).
1000s	In Constantinople, physician Simeon Seth stated that drinking to excess causes an inflammation in the liver. Arabic physician Muhammad Rhazes wrote, "Great damage is done by wine when abused and used regularly to get drunk."
1100s	Viking sagas speak of drinking matches to celebrate victories, alliances, and initiations. Distillation was used in the early Christian era and during the Middle Ages for various manufacturing purposes.
1300–1650	In medieval England, much brewing was done by women at home or in taverns. Many or most adult women were adept at brewing. The alewife, or female tavern keeper, was parodied as an ugly harridan, a flirtatious temptress, or even a blasphemous organizer of a mock mass who is condemned to hell, where she consorts with demons. *Piers Plowman*, written in the late 1300s by William Langland, is one notable example of such a narrative.
1390	In Geoffrey Chaucer's *The Canterbury Tales*, the Miller accounts for his muddled speech in telling his tale to drinking too much ale: "I am dronke...and therefore if that I mispeke or say: Wite it the ale of Southwark, I you pray." (Southwark was a major brewing center). During the late 1300s, much beer was manufactured and exported from the Netherlands to England and France; this manufacture and trade peaked around 1400.
1400s	Distillation devices were used in Sweden.
early 1500s	In England, until the reign of Henry VIII, monasteries were centers of brewing excellence and supported themselves through sales of beer. Henry broke this system up, and thus the

	secular brewing industry experienced a boom. An early trend developed of brewing beer with hops from the Netherlands. This was a period of high alcohol consumption, though hops were banned for several decades, denounced as a "Protestant plant."
1552	In reaction to widespread drunkenness and its ill effects on society, it became a civil offense in England. Inebriates were paraded through town wearing a beer barrel, known as the "drunkard's cloak." Laws were enacted to limit the number of taverns in a given town.
1500s	Distilled drinks were consumed in Europe. France witnessed the rising popularity of the cabaret.
1592	Elizabethan writer Thomas Nash observed that there were eight "species" of drunkenness, a terminology not used again for 360 years, when alcoholism researcher E.M. Jellinek cited Nash and used Greek letters to distinguish alcoholism species.
1600s	*Genever*, nicknamed gin, was distilled in the Netherlands and was introduced into England by mid-century.
1622	The Reverend Samuel Ward writes "Woe to Drunkards." Preachers of this time refer to drunkenness as a progressive addiction.
1630	A group of Puritans landed at the Massachusetts Bay Colony with 10,000 gallons of beer.
1662	John Winthrop, governor of Connecticut, brewed beer from Indian corn.
1600s	British colonists in America turned from traditional beer to distilled spirits such as rum and brandy, including rum that was 150 proof, or 75 percent alcohol. The first distillery in the colonies opened in Boston in 1700.
early 1700s	British colonists in America distilled cider into applejack and pears into perry. In the southern colonies, peaches were distilled into brandy.
1730–1751	A gin "epidemic" broke out in London. William Hogarth, a major English painter, printmaker, and social critic, satirized the evils of the consumption of gin as a contrast to the merits of drinking beer in his engraving *Gin Lane*.
1750s	Future U.S. president John Adams expressed concern over "spirituous liquors" and over taverns that he called "dens of iniquity." Later, independence from Great Britain was debated and planned in taverns, and liberty poles were erected in front of many taverns. The British authorities considered taverns hotbeds of sedition.
1784	Benjamin Rush, a signer of the Declaration of Independence, published "An Inquiry into the Effects of Ardent Spirits on the Human Mind and Body." In the document, he broke

with mainstream opinion in denying the health benefits of alcohol, catalogued a series of medical conditions caused by intemperate drinking, and recommended switching to beer and wine. But it was not until the 1810s that most medical writers began to change their view of alcohol as fortifying and healthy and adopt a negative view of alcohol as poison. He stated that stated that habitual drunkenness was a symptom of a mental obsession and that craving was set off by drunkenness itself.

1789   Bourbon was first produced in Kentucky.

1790–1840s Office seekers thought it necessary to treat the electorate with liquor during political campaigns, even at polling places, as a reward for making the long trek to hear speeches and vote.

1790s   George Washington opened a large whiskey distillery at Mount Vernon, and hundreds of distilleries opened during this decade. Whiskey started to supplant rum as the alcoholic beverage of choice. The building of a system of roads necessitated resting places and the means of changing horses, and the tavern and inn flourished as an institution for stagecoach travelers and freight and mail carriers. These venues functioned as centers of information, entertainment, and sociability—as locations for political argument, tavern games, and singing of ballads, and as places for musicians and artists to hold forth.

1791   At Alexander Hamilton's request, the U.S. Congress approved an excise tax on spirit distillers. He argued that the distilling industry was one of the most "mature" industries in the nation and could therefore bear the tax burden. He tacked on a "moral function" for the tax that higher prices would reduce alcohol consumption. The Internal Revenue Service was created to carry out the tax system.

1792   Distillers were mostly Appalachian frontier farmers in isolated underdeveloped areas—one-fourth of distilleries were in western Pennsylvania—where whiskey was actually a form of currency. The whiskey tax cut into their currency and caused hardship, so distillers in Pennsylvania and North Carolina withheld their payments and skirmished with authorities, roughing up tax agents.

1794   The Whiskey Rebellion came to a head in July when a federal marshal was attacked in Allegheny County, Pennsylvania. Elsewhere in the state, the residence of a regional inspector was burned, and mobs rioted in Pittsburgh. On August 7, President Washington called out a militia of 13,000 and personally led the troops to suppress the uprising. This was the first test of power of the new federal government, which asserted its right to enforce order in one state with troops from other states.

1800	President Jefferson abolished all internal taxes, including the whiskey excise tax and the land tax.
	Among the Seneca Indians in upstate New York, many of whom were depressed and drinking heavily, the prophet Handsome Lake had a series of visions that led to promotion of a mixture of Native American and Christian theology that promoted cultural revitalization, economic progress, and temperance.
1800–1830	Alcohol use, constructed as a social problem in America, is seen as a cause of disorder, ill health, sinfulness, family disintegration, and a lack of social progress. The founding of the temperance movement during the years 1808–1813 is connected to other themes of social improvement and to the wave of religious revival known as the Second Great Awakening.
1800–1900	Alcohol misuse variously described as a vice, sin, moral weakness or disease, or a vice or sin that develops into a true disease when it is out of control.
1804	Scottish physician Thomas Trotter stated that "the habit of drunkenness is a disease of the mind."
1810	Benjamin Rush called for an "asylum for inebriates," or a "sober house."
1813	Delerium tremens, which occurs during severe withdrawal from alcohol, is described in British medical journals.
1820–1840s	Temperance politics were first tied to African American churches and the Abolitionist movement. The African Methodist Episcopal Zion Church strongly supported both issues. Later, Fredrick Douglass proclaimed, "It was as well to be a slave to master, as to be a slave to whiskey and rum. When a slave was drunk, the slaveholder had no fear that he would plan an insurrection, no fear that he would escape to the North. It was the sober, thinking slave who was dangerous, and needed the vigilance of his master to keep him a slave." Holidays, when liquor was permitted, were to Douglass a cruel escape valve that encouraged frivolity and passivity.
1826	Lyman Beecher's Six Sermons on Intemperance contributed to the temperance movement.
1830	At the high point in consumption of alcohol in the United States, Americans consumed 7.1 gallons of absolute alcohol per capita. The average American male drank half a pint of hard liquor per day, binge drinking rose among males, and drinking occurred at any time of day and at any event. Women, however, tended to drink alcohol-based "medications" and "cordials" in public, though privately, they drank alcoholic beverages at home. Some people at the time considered the United States "a nation of drunkards."

1831	The American Temperance Society reported that two million people renounced liquor, and temperance societies reported 1.5 million members.
1832	Scottish physician Robert Macnish published *Anatomy of Drunkenness*, which included descriptions of seven types of drunkards: "the sanguineous drunkard, the melancholy drunkard, the surly drunkard, the phlegmatic drunkard, the nervous drunkard, the choleric drunkard, and the periodic drunkard."
1833	Richard "Dicky" Turner used the word *teetotaler* in a temperance speech.
1840	Opponents of presidential candidate William Henry Harrison said the "old man would be better off in a log cabin, with a jug." This attempt at defamation backfired; Harrison handed out small bottles of hard cider to solidify his populist image and won easily.
1840–60	Large-scale Irish and German immigration occurred in the United States; the newcomers did not share the temperance philosophy.
1842	The Sons of Temperance was founded.
1844	This year marked the rise and fall of the Washingtonians, an early working-class recovery fellowship that at one point had 200,000 adherents. Meetings featured the "experience speech," during which reformed drunkards spoke of their struggle with alcohols. This approach predated Alcoholics Anonymous.
1845	As a result of the wide range of temperance movements and organizations, the amount of alcohol drunk by the average American fell from 7.1 gallons per capita to 1.8 gallons in this year.
1849	Swedish physician Magnus Huss coins the term *alcoholism* in his influential book *Alcoholismus Chronicus*. At the time, many diseases ended in "-ism."
1850s	The first wave of prohibitionist activity occurred in the United States. A prohibition law was enacted in Maine in 1851. By 1855, 12 additional states passed the so-called Maine laws.
1850s–1865	Most of the Maine laws failed to be implemented or were reversed as the nation's focus turned to the conflict between North and South. The revenue from federal taxes on liquor was crucial to the nation and the war effort. Associations of liquor dealers were effective in countering prohibitionism, and a culture of drinking revived in the army and among the new waves of immigrants.
1850s–1900	The urban saloon, associated in the minds of opponents as a hotbed of sin became prominent, and "blind pigs," or unlicensed saloons, proliferated. During the last two decades

of the century, many brewers and liquor manufacturers sponsored saloons.

1858	The New York State Inebriate Asylum, in Binghamton, was the first institution built, funded, and designed to treat alcoholism as a mental disorder.
1872	The Drunkards Club in New York City, an early recovery fellowship like the Sons of Temperance and the Washingtonians, was founded.
1873	The Woman's Christian Temperance Union was founded under the leadership of Frances Willard. Many WCTU leaders were also advocates for women's suffrage.
1881	Karl Wernicke, a German neurologist and psychiatrist, and S. S. Korsakoff, a Russian psychiatrist, separately describe alcoholic syndromes affecting the brain, today known as Wernicke-Korsakoff syndrome.
1880s	Suffragists such as Carry Nation and Frances Willard were active in the temperance and prohibition movements.
1884	At a New York campaign rally for James Blaine, the Republican Party candidate for president, Samuel Bouchard declared, "We are Republicans, and don't propose to leave our party and identify with the party whose antecedents have been rum, Romanism, and rebellion," managing to lump together supporters of liquor and Catholicism as well as the Confederacy during the Civil War. This comment backfired and galvanized the campaign of Democratic Party candidate Grover Cleveland, who then swept New York State and won the presidency.
1890	Jacob Riis, a Danish American photographer and social reformer, decried the evils of the saloon. There were 150,000 saloons in 1880 in the United States and 300,000 in 1900. The saloon was integrated into urban machine politics: It was a political gathering place and even a polling station. It also served as a social club, a place to play cards, read a newspaper, receive mail or make a telephone call, and use a bathroom. Complementary buffets were served 1890.
1896	The formation of the Anti-Saloon League signaled a new wave of prohibitionist politics. Two opposing movements, Wet and Dry, formed around the controversy over prohibiting alcohol. Drys were predominantly Protestant and rural, Southern, and Midwestern. Wets were more urban and ethnic and immigrant (Irish, Italian, German, and so on). Prohibition politics were more single issue, not tied into social movements such as suffragism or abolitionism, as they had been earlier in the 19th century.
1899	Carry Nation, an extremist within the WCTU, organized her saloon-raiding "hachetation" campaign.

1907–1919	Thirty-four states passed prohibition laws.
1913	The idea of a national prohibition amendment took shape.
1917	Congress passed the 18th Amendment to the Constitution, which effectively prohibited the sale and consumption of alcohol.
1919	The states ratified the 18th Amendment. The Volstead Act (formally the National Prohibition Act), named for Andrew Volstead, chairman of the House Judiciary Committee and the legislation's sponsor and facilitator, implemented the 18th Amendment. (The Anti-Saloon League's Wayne Wheeler actually drafted the language of the bill.) President Wilson vetoed it, but Congress immediately overrode his veto on October 28. A key phrase from the legislation read, "No person shall manufacture, sell, barter, transport, import, export, deliver, or furnish any intoxicating liquor except as authorized by this act."
1920	In January, Prohibition went into effect. Speakeasies and bootlegging immediately spread, and doctors and druggists prescribed whiskey, as well as patent medicines with high concentrations of alcohol.
1920s	Norms and values concerning alcohol use loosened during the so-called Roaring Twenties as people gravitated to speakeasies and clandestine cocktail parties; sex-segregated drinking declined. (Many cocktails were invented during this period.) Bootlegging became a major underground economy. A colony of heavy-drinking American expatriate writers known as the Lost Generation lived in Paris, and that subculture resonated with bohemian Americans. Half of the famous authors of the 20th century with reputations for heavy drinking were born just before the turn of the century and came of age in that era.
late 1920s–early 1930s	Lawlessness, gang wars over bootlegging turf, and corruption in law enforcement were common. Al "Scarface" Capone of Chicago made millions from bootlegging until convicted of tax evasion in 1931.

A movement supporting the repeal of Prohibition developed. Paradoxically, liberated women of the flapper era were active in repeal politics, as they had been earlier in prohibition politics. By 1933, the Women's Organization for National Prohibition Reform, claimed 1.5 million members; it joined the Association Against the Prohibition Amendment.

As proposed by newly inaugurated president Franklin D. Roosevelt, the Volstead Act was modified to permit 3.2 percent beer. On December 5, as a result of passage of the Blaine Act, the 21st Amendment was ratified, repealing Prohibition. This

	was a unique event, as no constitutional amendment before or since has been repealed.
1935	John D. Rockefeller supported the Council for Moderation. Members of the evangelical Christian organization the Oxford Group, led by Frank Buchman, William Griffiths Wilson, and Robert Smith, met in Akron, Ohio. Alcoholics Anonymous was founded on June 10. AA organizers developed a small "alcoholic squad" in the Oxford Group but broke away during 1937–39. The Twelve Steps and Twelve Traditions of AA and its basic text are developed.
1937–1938	The Research Council on Problems of Alcohol was founded.
1939	Marty Mann became the first woman in AA. She helped start the Yale School of Alcohol Studies (now at Rutgers) and organized the National Council on Alcoholism (now the National Council on Alcoholism and Drug Dependence, or NCADD).
	The basic AA text *Alcoholics Anonymous* was published. Alcoholism was described as "cunning, baffling, powerful," a progressive illness that affects victims' mental, physical, and spiritual health.
1940	The Yale Center for Alcohol Studies was founded by E. M. Jellinek and Mark Keller, and the quarterly *Journal of Studies on Alcohol* was first published.
1944	Marty Mann founded the National Committee on Education about Alcoholism.
	The Yale Center pioneered outpatient treatment of alcoholism.
1951	Al-Anon Family Groups were founded by Lois Wilson, wife of AA founder Bill W., and Ann Smith.
mid-1950s	The hybrid Minnesota Model of alcoholism treatment was developed, combining multidisciplinary professional care with the concepts of AA. Detoxification over the course of 2 to 7 days was followed by 28 days of inpatient care with individual and group therapy and didactic educational sessions, followed by outpatient aftercare. Recovering alcoholics functioned as counselors, marking the beginnings of the alcoholism-counseling profession.
mid-1950s–1970	With the second wave of African American migration north, rates of alcoholic liver disease, traditionally lower in black communities, doubled.
1960	E. M. Jellinek published *The Disease Concept of Alcoholism*. Following the AA approach, he defined alcoholism as a chronic, progressive disease, and he described the phases of alcoholism.
1967	The American Medical Society on Alcoholism, developed from the pioneering New York City Medical Society on

Alcoholism, was founded; it was later renamed the American Society on Addiction Medicine.

Congress passed the Comprehensive Alcoholism Prevention and Treatment Act, also known as the Hughes Act because it was championed by self-proclaimed recovering alcoholic Harold Hughes, chair of the U.S. Senate Subcommittee on Alcohol and Narcotics. The act created a federal infrastructure on alcohol treatment and prevention, required states to develop alcohol authorities, authorized development of the National Institute on Alcohol Abuse and Alcoholism (NIAAA) within the National Institutes of Health (NIH), and provided a large stimulus, in the form of grant awards, to the growth of alcoholism treatment. The insurance industry began to reimburse alcoholism treatment. From 1973 to 1977, the number of alcoholism-treatment programs increased from 500 to 2,400.

1972   The National Council on Alcoholism, later called the NCAAD, published "Criteria for the Diagnosis of Alcoholism."

1973   Vernon Johnson, an Episcopal priest and a recovered alcoholic who devoted his life to alcohol intervention, published *I'll Quit Tomorrow*, which introduced the concept of planned, formal intervention by family, friends, and employers to get alcoholics into treatment.

1974–1976   The reauthorization of the Hughes Act placed the NIAAA within the federal Alcohol, Drug Abuse, and Mental Health Administration (ADAMHA).

1975   Sociologist Jean Kirkpatrick, a recovered alcoholic, founded Women for Sobriety, an alternative to AA.

late 1970s Credentialing of alcoholism counselors with educational and work experience requirements developed in many states. At this time, alcohol and drug treatment were entirely separate, as were credentialing systems.

late 1970s–
early 1980s Participation in recovery programs passed from being a secret shame to being considered an open, proud achievement. The Betty Ford Institute, Fair Oaks Hospital, and Hazelden had prominent and rich clients that influenced this shift.

1980   Mothers Against Drunk Driving was founded by Cindy Lightner after her daughter was killed by a drunk driver. MADD has had a significant impact on public health and the reduction in drunken driving fatalities (by half) as well as changing public attitudes toward that behavior, formerly seen as normal.

1980s   An explosive growth of private, for-profit treatment facilities, from 295 in 1982 to 1,401 in 1990, occurred. The number of patients in alcoholism treatment rose from about a quarter million in 1982 to 1.8 million in 1991. It has been said that this was a period of profiteering by the alcoholism business.

1980s Microbreweries and craft breweries proliferated in the United States.

1983 The American Society on Alcoholism and Drug Dependencies (later called the American Society for Addiction Medicine, or ASAM) was founded.

mid–1980s The Adult Children of Alcoholics movement developed.

1986 Rational Recovery (RR), largely based on rational-emotive behavior therapy, an approach developed by Albert Ellis, was founded by social worker Jack Trimpey as an alternative to AA. It is a source of counseling, guidance, and direct instruction on self-recovery from addiction to alcohol and other drugs through planned, permanent abstinence.

1988 The American Medical Association recognized ASAM as a medical-specialty organization.

1989 Managed-care research showed that inpatient care is not necessary for a majority of alcoholics, and an insurance backlash against residential inpatient rehabilitation over the next ten years resulted in closure of over half of traditional rehabilitation facilities. Reimbursement for inpatient treatment declined from 28 days to 5 to 7 days. This change prompted the expansion of outpatient care as well as a new modality: intensive outpatient care.

1990 Founding of the International Coalition for Addictions Studies Education, an association of addictions educators in higher education. The coalition held its first national conference in 1994.

1991 ASAM published its Patient Placement Criteria as a rational plan for putting alcoholics and drug addicts into appropriate levels of care based on the severity of their syndrome. These levels of care ranged from outpatient care to intensive outpatient, residential, and hospital treatment.

1993 The Substance Abuse and Mental Health Services Administration founded the Addiction Technology Transfer Network to "bring science to service."

1994 SMART Recovery, an alternative to AA, was founded to emphasize a self-empowerment and self-reliance approach to treatment by helping recovering alcoholics manage thoughts, behavior, and emotions.

2000 Federal legislation compelled states to lower driving-while-intoxicated blood-alcohol levels to .08 percent (8/100 of 1%).

2000–2011 Spread of the Recovery Oriented System of Care paradigm of alcoholism treatment. This includes long-term "recovery monitoring" by recovery mentors, open public advocacy for treatment and prevention by recovering alcoholics, recognition of the recovery potential within all alcoholics, and a strengths-based, empowering approach to recovery.

2010   Federal government deliberates on combining the National Institute on Drug Abuse and National Institute on Alcohol Abuse and Alcoholism.

Federal ban on popular caffeinated malt beverages such as Four Loko.

2011   Addictions educators and counselors form the National Addiction Studies Accreditation Commission, similar to accreditation commissions for social work and counseling psychology curricula.

REFERENCES

Abbey, A. (2002). Alcohol-related sexual assault: A common problem among college student ts. *Journal of Studies on Alcohol and Drugs* (Suppl. 14), 118–128.

Abbey, A., Zawacki, T., & McAuslan, P. (2000). Alcohol and sexual perception. *Journal of Studies on Alcohol and Drugs, 61,* 688–697.

Abbey, A., Zawacki, R., Buck, P. O., Clinton, A. M., & McAuslan, P. (2001). Alcohol and sexual assault. *Alcohol Research and Health, 25*(1), 43–51.

ABC Online. (2010, July 14). Heatwave and vodka: A deadly Russian mix. Retrieved from http://abcnews.go.com/International/russia-heat-wave-vodka-deadly-mix-drowning/story?id=11170454

Addolorato, G., Caputo, F., Capristo, E., Domenicali, M., Bernardi, M., Janiri, L., Agabio, R.,...Gasbarrini, G. (2002). Baclofen efficacy in reducing alcohol craving and intake: A preliminary double-blind randomized controlled study. *Alcohol and Alcoholism, 37*(5), 504–508.

Al-Anon. (2011). *Al-Anon's path to recovery.* Retrieved from http://www.al-anon.alateen.org/pdf/S67.pdf

Al-Anon & Alateen. (2010). *Detachment.* Baltimore, MD: Al-Anon and Alateen. Retrieved from http://www.alanon-maryland.org/literature/detachment.php

Albalate, D. (2008). Lowering blood alcohol content levels to save lives: The European experience. *Journal of Policy Analysis and Management, 27*(1), 20–39.

Alcohol Policy Information System (2010). Retrieved from http://www.alcohol policy.niaaa.nih.gov/Home.html

Alcoholics Anonymous. (1976). *Alcoholics Anonymous.* AA General Service Office: Author.

Alibrandi, L. A. (1985). The folk psychotherapy of Alcoholics Anonymous. In S. Zimberg, J. Wallace, & S. B. Blume (Eds.), *Practical approaches to alcoholism psychotherapy* (2nd ed., pp. 239–257). New York: Plenum Press.

American Academy of Pediatrics (2010). *Policy statement—Alcohol use by youth and adolescents: A pediatric concern.* Retrieved from http://pediatrics.aap publications.org/cgi/reprint/peds.2010-0438v1

American Psychological Association (2000). *Diagnostic and statistical manual of mental disorders* (4th ed., text revision). Washington, DC: Author.

American Psychological Association (2010a). *303.90 alcohol dependence.* Retrieved from http://www.dsm5.org/ProposedRevisions/Pages/proposedre vision.aspx?rid=36#

American Psychological Association (2010b). *Substance-use disorder.* Retrieved from http://www.dsm5.org/ProposedRevisions/Pages/proposedrevision. aspx?rid=431#

American Society for Addiction Medicine. (2001). *American Society for Addiction Medicine patient placement criteria for the treatment of substance-related disorders, PPC 2-R.* Chevy Chase, MD: Author.

Andreasen, N. C. (1999). Understanding the causes of schizophrenia. *New England Journal of Medicine, 340*(8), 645–647.

Anton, R. F., O'Malley, S. S., Ciraulo, D. A., Cisler, R. A., Couper, D., Donovan, D. M., Gartfriend, D. R., Johnson, B. A. et al. (2006). Combined pharmacotherapies and behavioral interventions for alcohol dependence—The COMBINE study: A randomized controlled trial. *JAMA, 295,* 2003–2017.

Armstrong, E. M., & Abel, E. L. (2000). Fetal alcohol syndrome: The origins of a moral panic. *Alcohol and Alcoholism, 35*(3), 276–282.

Ausabel, D. (2002). *Theory and problems of adolescent development* (3rd ed.). New York: Writers Club Press.

Babor, T. F. (1992). Cross-cultural research on alcohol: A quoi bon? In J. E. Helzer & G. J. Canino (Eds.), *Alcoholism in North America, Europe, and Asia* (pp. 33–52). New York: Oxford University Press.

Babor, T. F., McRee, B. G., Kassebaum, P. A., Grimaldi, P. L., Ahmed, K., & Bray, J. (2007). Screening, brief intervention, and referral to treatment (SBIRT): Toward a public health approach to the management of substance abuse. *Substance Abuse: Journal of the Association for Medical Education and Research in Substance Abuse, 28*(3), 7–30.

Baez, A. (2005). Alcohol use among Dominican Americans: An explanation. In M. Delgado (Ed.), *Latino and alcohol use/misuse revisited* (pp. 53–65). Binghamton, NY: Haworth Press.

Bahr, S. J., & Hoffmann, J. P. (2010). Parenting style, religiosity, peers, and adolescent heavy drinking. *Journal of Studies on Alcohol and Drugs, 71*(4), 539–543.

Bahr, N., & Pendegast, D. (2007). *The millennial adolescent.* Camberwell, Australia: ACER Press.

Baum, D. (2003). Jake leg: How the blues diagnosed a medical mystery. *New Yorker, 79,* 50–57.

Bean, M. (1978). Denial and the psychological complications of alcoholism. In M. H. Bean & N. Zimberg (Eds.), *Dynamic approaches to the understanding and treatment of alcoholism* (pp. 55–96). New York: The Free Press.

Beck, A. T., Wright, F. D., Newman, C. F., & Liese, B. S. (1993). *Cognitive therapy of substance abuse.* New York: The Guilford Press.

Beckwith, C. (1993). The Jagerettes: Exploitative campus alcohol marketing. Campus Consortium. *Alliance of Higher Education Drug Prevention Consortium, 1*(1), 3.

Beerman, K. A., Smith, M. M., & Hall, R. L. (1988). Predictors of recidivism in DUIIs. *Journal of Studies on Alcohol, 49,* 443–449.

Bell, R. G. (1963). Comment on the article by D. L. Davies. *Quarterly Journal of Studies on Alcohol, 24,* 321–322.

Beman, D. S. (1995). Risk factors leading to adolescent substance abuse. *Adolescence, 20*(117), 201–208.

Bischof, G., Rumpf, H-J., Meyer, J., Hapke, U., & Ulrich, J. (2007). Stability of subtypes of natural recovery from alcohol dependence after two years. *Addiction, 102*(6), 904–908.

Black, C. (2002). *It will never happen to me: Growing up with addiction as youngsters, adolescents, adults* (2nd ed.). Center City, MN: Hazelden.

Blane, H. T. (1977). Acculturation and drinking in an Italian-American community. *Journal of Studies on Alcohol, 38,* 1324–1346.

Block, L. (2004). Health policy: What it is and what it does. In C. Harrington & C. Estes (Eds.), *Health policy: Crisis and reform in the U.S. health care delivery system* (4th ed., pp. 27–29). Sudbury, MA: Jones and Bartlett.

Blow, F. C. (2000). Substance abuse among older adults: An invisible epidemic. In F. C. Blow (Ed.), *Substance abuse among older adults: A treatment protocol.* Rockville, MD: Substance Abuse and Mental Health Services Administration. Executive Summary and Recommendations. Retrieved from http://www.ncbi.nlm.nih.gov/books/NBK26263/

Blum, D. (2010, February 19). The chemist's war: The little-told story of how the U.S. government poisoned alcohol during Prohibition with deadly consequences. *Slate.* Retrieved from http://www.slate.com/id/2245188

Blum, K., Chen, A.L-C., Braverman, E. R., Comings, D. E., Chen, T.J.H., Arcuri, V., Blum, S. H.,...Oscar-Berman, M. (2008). Attention deficit-hyperactivity disorder and reward deficiency syndrome. *Neuropsychiatric Disease and Treatment, 4*(5), 893–918.

Blum, K., & Payne, J. E. (1991). *Alcohol and the addictive brain.* New York: Free Press.

Blumberg, L. U., & Pittman, W. L. (1991). *Beware the first drink!: The Washingtonian Temperance Movement and Alcoholics Anonymous.* Seattle: Glen Abbey Books.

Borsari, B. E., & Carey, K. B. (1999). Understanding fraternity drinking: Five recurring themes in the literature, 1980–1998. *Journal of American College Health, 48*(1), 30–37.

Boudewyns, P. A., Woods, M. G., Hyer, L. A., & Albrecht, J. (1991). Chronic combat-related PTSD and concurrent substance abuse: Implications for treatment of this frequent "dual diagnosis." *Journal of Traumatic Stress, 4*(4), 549–560.

Bradford, B., Karnitsching, J., Powell, L., & Garbutt, J. (2007). Rates of ethanol metabolism decrease in sons of alcoholics following a priming dose of ethanol. *Alcohol, 41*(4), 263–270.

Brennan, P. L., Schutte, K. K., & Moos, R. F. (2010). Retired status and older adults' 10-year drinking trajectories. *Journal of Studies on Alcohol and Drugs, 71*(2), 169–179.

Breslow, R. A., Faden, V. B., & Smothers, B. (2003). Alcohol consumption by elderly Americans. *Journal of Studies on Alcohol, 64,* 884–892.

Brick, J. (2008). *Handbook of the medical consequences of alcohol and drug abuse* (2nd ed.). New York: Routledge.

Brister, H. A., Wetherill, R. R., & Fromme, K. (2010). Anticipated versus actual alcohol consumption during 21st birthday celebrations. *Journal of Studies on Alcohol and Drugs, 71*(2), 180–183.

Brodsky, A., & Peele, S. (1991, November). *Reason*, pp. 34–39. Stanton Peele Addiction Web site. Retrieved from http://www.peele.net/lib/aaabuse.html

Bronisch, T., & Wittchen, H-U. (1992). Lifetime and 6-month prevalence of abuse and dependence of alcohol in the Munich follow-up study. *European Archives of Psychiatry and Clinical Neuroscience, 241*(5), 273–282.

Brown, J., Conte, J. J., Foxx, J., Henderson, C., Melancon, B., Naim, F., Nash, T, … Walker, N. (2009). Blame it on the Goose. Licensed by Gracenote Lyrics. Performed by Jamie Foxx.

Brown, J. M., Council, C. L., Penne, M. A., & Gfroerer, J. C. (2005). Immigrants and 385 substance: Findings from the 1990–2001 National Survey on Drug Use and Health. Retrieved from http://www.oas.samhsa.gov/immigrants/immigrants.pdf

Buckland, P. R. (2008). Will we ever find the genes for addiction? *Addiction, 103*(11), 1768–1776.

Burk, J., & Sher, K. (1990). Labeling the child of an alcoholic: Negative stereotyping by mental health professionals and peers. *Journal of Studies on Alcohol and Drugs, 51,* 156–163.

Burke, B. L., Arkowitz, H., & Menchola, M. (2003). The efficacy of motivational interviewing: A meta-analysis of controlled clinical trials. *Journal of Consulting and Clinical Psychology, 71*(5), 843–861.

Burns, T. F. (1980). Getting rowdy with the boys. *Journal of Drug Issues, 10,* 273–286.

Burroughs, A. (2003). *Dry.* New York: Picador.

Caetano, R., & Herd, D. (1984). Black drinking practices in northern California. *American Journal of Drug and Alcohol Abuse, 10*(4), 571–587.

Campbell, A. (1991). *The girls in the gang* (2nd ed.). New Brunswick, NJ: Rutgers University Press.

Cashin, J. R., Presley, C. A., & Meilman, P. W. (1998). Alcohol use in the Greek system: Follow the leader? *Journal of Studies on Alcohol, 59*(1), 63–70.

Caudill, B. D., Crosse, S. B., Campbell, B., Howard, J., Luckey, B., & Blane, H. T. (2006). High-risk drinking among college fraternity members: A national perspective. *Journal of American College Health, 55*(3), 141–155.

Cavaiola, A., & Wuth, C. (2002). *Assessment and treatment of the DUI offender.* New York: Haworth Press.

Center for Substance Abuse Treatment. (1993). *Center for Substance Abuse Treatment: Levels of care.* Retrieved from http://www.ncbi.nlm.nih.gov/books/NBK25846/

Center for Substance Abuse Treatment. (1995). *TIP 11: Simple screening instruments for alcohol and other substance abuse disorders and infectious diseases.* Retrieved from http://www.ncbi.nlm.nih.gov/books/NBK14945/

Center for Substance Abuse Treatment. (1999). *Enhancing motivation for change in substance abuse treatment.* Rockville, MD: Substance Abuse and Mental Health Services Administration. Retrieved from http://www.ncbi.nlm.nih.gov/books/bv.fcgi?rid=hstat5.chapter.61302

Centers for Disease Control and Prevention. (2003). Fetal alcohol syndrome—South Africa. *Morbidity and Mortality Weekly Report, 52*(28), 660–662.

Centers for Disease Control and Prevention. (2008, August 29). Alcohol-attributable deaths and years of potential life lost among American Indians and Alaska Natives—United States, 2001–2005. *Morbidity and Mortality Weekly Report.*

Centers for Disease Control and Prevention. (2011). *Fetal Alcohol Spectrum Disorder/Data.* Retrieved from http://www.cdc.gov/ncbddd/fasd/data.html

Cervantes, R. C., Salgado de Snyder, V. N., & Padilla, A. M. (1989). Posttraumatic stress in immigrants from Cental America and Mexico. *Hospital and Community Psychiatry, 40,* 615–619.

Chalfont, H. P., & Beckley, R. E. (1977). Beguiling and betraying: the image of alcohol use in country music. *Journal of Studies of Alcohol and Drugs, 38*(7), 445–451.

Cheever, S. (1999). *Note found in a bottle—My life as a drinker.* New York: Washington Square Press.

Choose Responsibility. (2011). Breeds disrespect for law and causes ethical compromises. Retrieved from http://www.chooseresponsibility.org/article/view/15541/1/2642/

Christopher, J. (1988). *How to stay sober: Recovery without religion.* Amherst, NY: Prometheus Books.

Christopher, J. (1989). *Unhooked: Staying sober and drug-free.* Amherst, NY: Prometheus Books.

Chudley, A. E. (2008). Fetal alcohol spectrum disorder: Counting the invisible—mission impossible? *Archives of Disease in Childhood, 93,* 721–722.

Coles, C. D., & Platzman, K. A. (1993). Behavioral development in children prenatally exposed to drugs and alcohol. *International Journal of the Addictions, 28,* 1393–1433.

Connors, G. J., & Alpher, V. S. (1989). Alcohol themes within country-western songs. *International Journal of the Addictions, 24,* 445–451.

Core Institute. (2005). *2005 statistics on alcohol and other drug use on American campuses.* Carbondale, IL: Core Institute.

Corte, C., & Zucker, R. A. (2008). Self-concept disturbances: Cognitive vulnerability for early drinking and early drunkenness in adolescents at high risk for alcohol problems. *Addictive Behaviors, 33*(10), 1282–1290.

Coyhis, D. (2000). Culturally specific addiction recovery for Native Americans. In J. Krestan (Ed.), *Bridges to Recovery.* New York: Free Press.

Crawford, L. A., & Novak, K. B. (2006). Alcohol abuse as a rite of passage: The effect of beliefs about alcohol and the college experience on undergraduates' drinking behaviors. *Journal of Drug Education, 36*(3), 193–212.

Cremeens, J. L., Nelson, D., Naimi, T. S., Brewer, R. D., Pearson, W. S., & Chavez, P. R. (2009). Sociodemographic differences in binge drinking among adults—14 states. *Morbidity and Mortality Weekly Report, 58*(12), 301–304.

Crenshaw, T. L., & Goldberg, J. P. (1996). *Sexual pharmacology: Drugs that affect sexual function.* New York: Norton.

Cucchiaro, S., Ferreira, J., Jr., & Sicherman, A. (1974). *The effect of the 18-year-old drinking age on auto accidents.* Cambridge, MA: Massachusetts Institute of Technology Operations Research Center.

D'Avanzo, C. E., Frye, B., & Froman, R. (1994). Culture, stress and substance in Cambodian refugee women. *Journal of Studies on Alcohol and Drugs, 55,* 420–426.

Davies, D. L. (1962). Normal drinking in recovered alcohol addicts. *Quarterly Journal of Studies on Alcohol, 23*, 94–104.

Dawson, D. A. (2000). Beyond black, white, and Hispanic: Race, ethnic origin, and drinking patterns in the United States. *Journal of Substance Abuse, 10*(4), 321–339.

De Sousa, A. (2010). The pharmacotherapy of alcohol dependence: A state of the art review. *Psychopharmacology Today, 8*(1), 69–82.

De Tocqueville, A. (2000). *Democracy in America.* H. Mansfield & D. Winthrop (Trans., Eds.). Chicago: University of Chicago Press.

Demossier, M. (2005). Consuming wine in France. In T. M. Wilson (Ed.), *Drinking cultures* (pp. 129–154). Oxford: Berg.

Dennis, P. A. (1979). The role of the drunk in a Oaxacan village. In M. Marshall (Ed.), *Beliefs, Behavior, and Alcoholic Beverages* (pp. 54–64). Ann Arbor: University of Michigan Press.

Department of Justice. (2010). *Alcohol and crime: Data from 2002 to 2008.* Washington, DC: Author. Retrieved from http://bjs.ojp.usdoj.gov/index.cfm?ty=pbdetail&iid=2313

Dick, D. M., & Agrawal, A. (2008). The genetics of alcohol and other drug dependence. *Alcohol Research and Health, 31*(2), 111–118.

Diehl, A. D. (n.d.). Effects of alcohol on the liver. *Research Society on Alcoholism Lecture Series.* Retrieved from http://www.rsoa.org/lectures/2_07/index.html

Dill, P. L., & Wells-Parker, E. (2006). Court-mandated treatment for convicted drinking drivers. *Alcohol Research & Health, 29*(1), 41–48.

Ditter, S. M., Elder, R. W., Shults, R. A., Sleet, D. A., Compton, R., & Nichols, J. L. (2005). Effectiveness of designated driver programs for reducing alcohol-impaired driving: A systematic review. *American Journal of Preventive Medicine, 28*(5 Suppl), 280–287.

Doll, B., & Lyon, M. (1998). Risk and resilience: Implications for the delivery of mental health services in schools. *School Psychology Review, 27,* 348–363.

Dorris, M. (1989). *The broken cord.* New York: HarperCollins.

Douglass, R. L., Filkins, L. D., & Clark, F. A. (1974). *The effect of lower legal drinking ages on youth crash involvement.* Ann Arbor: University of Michigan Highway Safety Research Institute.

Drexel University. *Rites of Passage.* Retrieved from http://www.pages.drexel.edu/~ags25/mwebsites.htm

Ducci, F., & Goldman, D. (2008). Genetic approaches to addiction: Genes and alcohol. *Addiction, 103*(9), 1414–1428.

Earls, F., Reich, W., Jung, K. G., & Cloninger, C. R. (1988). Psychopathology in children of alcoholic and antisocial parents. *Alcoholism: Clinical and Experimental Research, 12,* 481–487.

Eber, C. (2000). *Women and alcohol in a highland Maya town.* Austin: University of Texas Press.

Edwards, J. T. (1990). *Treating chemically dependent families.* Minneapolis: Johnson Institute.

Egan, V., & Cordan, G. (2009). Barely legal: Perceptions of attraction and age as a function of make-up, sex, age of participant, and alcohol use. *British Journal of Psychology, 100,* 415–427. Retrieved from http://leicester.academia.edu/documents/0011/4626/Barely_legal_PDF__published_version_.pdf

Ellis, A., McInerney, J. F., DiGiuseppe, R., & Yeager, R. J. (1988). *Rational-emotive therapy with alcoholics and substance abusers.* Boston: Allyn and Bacon.

Eltner, S. L. (2010). Prevalence and correlates of at-risk drinking among older adults: The Project Share study. *Journal of General Internal Medicine, 25*(8), 840–846.

Emrick, C. D. (1987). Alcoholics Anonymous: Affiliation processes and effectiveness as treatment. *Alcoholism: Clinical and Experimental Research, 11,* 416–423.

Engs, R. (2000). *Clean living movements: American cycles of health reform.* Westport, CT: Praeger.

Enos, G. (2010, January 9). Massachusetts physician praises effects of Vivitrol. *Addiction Professional.* Online blog post.

Erikson, E. H. (1968). *Identity: Youth and crisis.* New York: Norton.

European Health Alliance (2010). WHO global strategy to reduce the harmful use of alcohol. Retrieved from http://www.epha.org/a/3878

Feeney, G. F., Connor, J. P., Young, R. M., Tucker, J., & McPherson, A. (2006). Combined acamprosate and naltrexone, with cognitive behavioural therapy is superior to either medication alone for alcohol abstinence: A single centre's experience with pharmacotherapy. *Alcohol Alcohol, 41*(3), 321–332.

Fergusson, D. M., Boden, J. M., & Horwood, L. J. (2009). Tests of causal links between alcohol abuse or dependence and major depression. *Archives of General Psychiatry, 66*(3), 260–266.

Finney, A. (2003). Alcohol and intimate partner violence: Key findings from the research. *Findings, 216.* London: British Home Office.

Fleming, M. S., Milic, N., & Harris, R. (2006). Ethanol. In L. Brunton et al. (Eds.), *The pharmacology basis of therapeutics* (11th ed., pp. 429–446). New York: McGraw-Hill.

Foran, H. M., & O'Leary, K. D. (2008). Problem drinking, jealousy, and anger control: Variables predicting physical aggression against a partner. *Journal of Family Violence, 23*(3), 141–148.

Ford, B. (1978). *The times of my life.* New York: HarperCollins.

Ford, B. (1987). *Betty: A glad awakening.* Garden City, NJ: Doubleday.

Ford, G. (2010). Alcohol abuse: The economic costs. Retrieved from http://www2. potsdam.edu/hansondj/controversies/1104197649.html

Fox, A. (2008). Sociocultural factors that foster or inhibit alcohol-related violence, in alcohol and violence: Exploring patterns and responses. Retrieved from http://ec.europa.eu/health/ph_determinants/life_style/alcohol/Forum/ docs/alcohol_lib18_en.pdf

Garbarino, A. J. (1971). Life in the city: Chicago. In J. O. Wadell & O. M. Watson (Eds.), *The American Indian in urban society* (pp. 168–205). Boston, MA: Little, Brown.

Garcia, V., & Gondolf, E. (2004). Transnational Mexican farmworkers and problem drinking: A review of the literature. *Contemporary Drug Problems, 31*(1), 129–164.

Garvey, P. (2005). Drunk and (dis)orderly: Norwegian drinking parties in the home. In T. W. Wilson (Ed.), *Drinking cultures.* Oxford: Berg.

Gelernter, J., Goldman, D., & Risch, N. (1993). The A1 allele at the D2 dopamine receptor gene and alcoholism: A reappraisal. *Journal of the American Medical Association, 269,* 1676.

George, W. H., & Martinez, L. (2002). Victim blaming in rape: Effects of victim and perpetrator race, type of rape, and participant racism. *Psychology of Women Quarterly, 26,* 110–119.

Gilbert, M. J. (1991). Acculturation and changes in drinking patterns among Mexican-American women. *Alcohol Research & Health, 15*(3), 234–238.

Glatt, M. (1958). Group therapy in alcoholism. *British Journal of Addiction, 54*(2), 133.

Goldman, M. S., & Roehrich, L. (1991). Alcohol expectancies and sexuality. *Alcohol Research & Health, 15,* 126–132.

Gordon, A. (1981). The cultural context of drinking and indigenous therapy for alcohol problems in three migrant Hispanic cultures. *Journal of Studies on Alcohol and Drugs* (Suppl. 9), 217–240.

Gorwood, P., Bellivier, F., Adès, J., & Leboyer, M. (2000). The DRD2 gene and the risk for alcohol dependence in bipolar patients. *European Psychiatry, 15*(2), 103–108.

Grant, B. F., & Dawson, D. A. (1997). Age at onset of alcohol use and its association with DSM-IV alcohol abuse and dependence: Results from the National
Longitudinal Alcohol Epidemiologic Survey. *Journal of Substance Abuse, 9,*
103–110.

Grant, B. F., Dawson, D. A., Stinson, F. S., Chou, S. P., Dufour, M. C., &
Pickering, R. P. (2006). The 12-month prevalence and trends in DSM-IV
alcohol abuse and dependence: United States, 1991–1992 and 2001–2002.
Alcohol Research & Health, 29(2), 79–91.

Gray, G. C., Kaiser, K. S., Hawksworth, A. W., Hall, F. W., & Barrett-Connor,
E. (1999). Increased postwar symptoms and psychological morbidity among
U.S. Navy Gulf War veterans. *American Journal of Tropical Medicine and
Hygiene, 60,* 758–766.

Greene, R. R. (2002). *Resiliency: An integrated approach to practice, policy, and
research.* Washington, DC: NASW Press.

Greenfield, L., & Henneberg, M. (2000, June 11–14). Alcohol, crime, and the
criminal justice system. Presented at the Alcohol and Crime: Research and
Practice for Prevention, Alcohol Policy XII Conference, Washington, DC.

Grob, C., & Dobkin de Rios, M. (1992). Adolescent drug use in cross-cultural
perspective. *Journal of Drug Issues, 22*(1), 121–138.

Hall, E. T. (1966). *The hidden dimension.* New York: Doubleday.

Hall, G. S. (1904). *Adolescence: Its psychology and its relations to physiology,
anthropology, sociology, sex, crime, religion, and education* (2 vols.). New
York: Appleton.

Hall, T. M. (2005). Pivo at the heart of Europe: Beer drinking and Czech identi-
ties. In *Drinking cultures.* Oxford: Bern.

Hamill, P. (1994). *A drinking life.* New York: Little, Brown.

Hanson, D. J. (1999). *The legal drinking age: Science vs. ideology.* Retrieved from
http://www2.potsdam.edu/hansondj/YouthIssues/1046348726.html

Harmon, A. (1998, April 30). On-line trail to an off-line killing. *The New York
Times,* A1.

Hartley, L. P. (1953). *The go-between.* New York: New York Review of Books
Classics.

Hasin, D. S., & Beseler, C. L. (2009). Dimensionality of lifetime alcohol abuse, dependence, and binge drinking. *Drug and Alcohol Dependence, 101,* 53–61.

Hasin, D. S., Paykin, A., Endicott, J., & Grant, B. (1999). The validity of DSM-IV
alcohol abuse: Drunk drivers vs. all others. *Journal on the Study of Alcohol,
60,* 746–755.

Hawkins, J. D., Catalano, R. F., & Arthur, M. (2002). Promoting science-based
prevention in communities. *Addictive Behaviors, 90*(5), 1–26.

Hawkins, J. D., Catalano, R. F., & Miller, J. Y. (1992). Risk and protective factors for
alcohol and other drug problems in adolescence and early adulthood: Implications for substance abuse prevention. *Psychological Bulletin, 112,* 64–105.

Hawkins, J. D., Lishner, D. M., Catalano, R. F., & Howard, M. O. (1986). Childhood
predictors of adolescent substance abuse: Toward an empirically grounded
theory. *Journal of Children in Contemporary Society, 18,* 11–48.

Hayashida, M., Alterman, A. I., McLellan, T., O'Brien, C. P., Purtill, J. J., Volpicelli, J. R., ... Hall, C. P. (1989). Comparative effectiveness and costs of inpatient and outpatient detoxification of patients with mild-to-moderate alcohol withdrawal syndrome. *The New England Journal of Medicine, 320*(6), 358–365.

Heath, D. B. (1975). A critical review of ethnographic studies of alcohol use. In R. J. Gibbons & Y. Israel (Eds.), *Research advances in alcohol and drug problems* (Vol. 2). New York: Wiley.

Heath, D. B. (2000). *Drinking occasions: Comparative perspectives on alcohol and culture.* New York: Taylor and Francis.

Herd, D. (1984). Ambiguity in black drinking norms: An ethnohistorical interpretation. In L. A. Bennett & G. M. Ames (Eds.), *The American experience with alcohol* (pp. 149–170). New York: Plenum Press.

Herd, D. (1985). Migration, cultural transformation, and the rise of black liver cirrhosis mortality. *Addiction, 80*(4), 397–410.

Hingson, R., Heeren, T., & Winter, M. (1996). Lowering state legal blood alcohol limits to 0.08%: The effect on fatal motor vehicle crashes. *Public Health Brief, 86*(9), 1297–1299.

Hingson, R. W., Heeren T., Zakocs, R. C., Kopstein, A., & Wechsler, H. (2002). Magnitude of alcohol-related mortality and morbidity among U.S. college students ages 18–24. *Journal of Studies on Alcohol and Drugs, 63,* 136–144.

Hingson, R. W., Zha, W., & Weitzman, E. R. (2009). Magnitude of and trends in alcohol-related mortality and morbidity among U.S. college students ages 18–24, 1998–2005. *Journal of Studies on Alcohol and Drugs* (Suppl. 16), 12–20.

Hoffman, J. (2009, August 16). A heroine of cocktail moms sobers up. *The New York Times,* Styles, p. 1.

Hoge, C. W., Castro, C. A., Messer, S. C., McGurk, D., Cotting, D. I., & Koffman, R. L. (2004). Combat duty in Iraq and Afghanistan, mental health problems, and barriers to care. *New England Journal of Medicine, 351,* 13–22.

Horowitz, H. L. (1987). *Campus life.* New York: Knopf.

Howland, J., & Hingson, R. (1987). Alcohol as a risk factor for injuries or death due to fires and burns: Review of the literature. *Public Health Reports, 102*(5), 475–483.

Humphreys, K. (2003). Alcohol & drug abuse: A research-based analysis of the moderation management controversy. *Psychiatric Services, 54,* 621–622.

Humphreys, K., Huebsch, P., Moos, R. H., & Suchinsky, R. T. (1999). Alcohol and drug abuse: The transformation of the Veterans Affairs substance abuse treatment system. *Psychiatric Services, 50,* 1399–1401.

Inaba, D. S., & Cohen, W. E. (1997). *Uppers, downers, all arounders* (6th ed.). Medford, OR: CNS Productions.

INCASE. (2011). International Coalition for Addiction Studies Education. Retrieved from http://www.incase-edu.net

Institute of Alcohol Studies. (2006). Economic costs and benefits. Retrieved from http://www.ias.org.uk/resources/factsheets/economic_costs_benefits.pdf

Institute of Medicine (Ed.). (1990). *Broadening the base of treatment for alcohol problems.* Report of a study by a committee of the Institute of Medicine, Division of Mental Health and Behavioral Medicine (pp. 30–31). Washington, DC: National Academies Press.

International Center for Alcohol Policies. (2010). Policy issues. Retrieved from http://www.icap.org/PolicyIssues/tabid/62/Default.aspx

International Center for Alcohol Policies. (2011). About ICAP. Retrieved from http://www.icap.org/AboutICAP/tabid/55/Default.aspx

Janis, I., & Mann, L. (1977). *Decision making: A psychological analysis of conflict, choice, and commitment.* New York: Free Press.

Jason, L. A., & Ferrari, J. R. (Eds.). (2009). Recovery from addiction in communal living settings: The Oxford House Model [Special Issue]. *Journal of Groups in Addiction & Recovery, 4*(1–2).

Jason, L. A., Olson, B. D., & Foli, K. (2008). *Rescued lives: The Oxford House approach to substance abuse.* New York: Routledge.

Jellinek, E. M. (1946). Phases in the drinking history of alcoholics: Analysis of a survey conducted by the official organ of Alcoholics Anonymous. *Journal of Studies on Alcohol and Drugs, 7,* 1–88.

Jellinek, E. M. (1960). *The disease concept of alcoholism.* New Haven, CT: Hillhouse.

Jennings, D. (2010, June 12). Bidding farewell to ghosts of pain. *The New York Times,* p. D5. Retrieved from http://well.blogs.nytimes.com/2010/06/21/bidding-farewell-to-ghosts-of-pain

Jilek, W. (1993). Traditional healing against alcoholism and drug dependence. *Curare, 16,* 145–160.

Johns Hopkins. (2010). *Alcoholic liver disease: Causes.* Baltimore, MD: Johns Hopkins Medicine, Gastroenterology and Hepatology. Retrieved from at http://www.hopkins-gi.org/GDL_Disease.aspx?CurrentUDV=31&GDL_Cat_ID=83F0F583-EF5A-4A24-A2AF-0392A3900F1D&GDL_Disease_ID=FE859301-360B-4201-959B-3256E859CD01

Johnson, P. B., Richter, L., Kleber, A., McClellan, T., & Carise, D. (2005). Telescoping of drinking-related behaviors: Gender, racial/ethnic, and age comparisons. *Substance Use & Misuse, 40*(8), 1139–1151.

Johnson, V. (1973). *I'll quit tomorrow.* New York: Harper and Row.

Johnson, V. (1986). *Intervention, how to help someone who doesn't want help: A step-by step guide for families and friends of chemically dependent persons.* Minneapolis: Johnson Institute Books.

Johnston, J., & McGovern, J. (2004). Alcohol related falls: An interesting pattern of injuries. *Emergency Medical Journal, 21,* 185–188.

Join Together. (2009). Horrific van crash highlights disturbing trend in female DUIs. Retrieved from http://www.jointogether.org/news/headlines/inthenews/2009/horrific-van-crash-highlights.html

Jones, B. T., Jones, B. C., Thomas, A., & Piper, J. (2003). Alcohol consumption increases attractiveness ratings of opposite-sex faces: A possible third route to risky sex. *Addiction, 98*(8), 1069–1075.

Jones, K. L., & Smith, D. W. (1973). Recognition of the fetal alcohol syndrome in early infancy. *Lancet, 2,* 999–1001.

Jones, N. E., Pieper, C. F., & Robertson, L. S. (1992). The effect of legal drinking age on fatal injuries of adolescents and young adults. *American Journal of Public Health, 82,* 112–115.

Karp, I. (1980). Beer drinking and social experience in an African society. In I. Karp & C. S. Bird (Eds.), *Explorations in African systems of thought.* Bloomington: Indiana University Press.

Kassel, J. D., & Wagner, E. F. (1993). Processes of change in Alcoholics Anonymous: A review of possible mechanisms. *Psychotherapy, 30*(2), 222–234.

Kendall, R. E. (1983). Alcohol and suicide. *Substance and Alcohol Actions/ Misuse, 4*(2–3), 121–127.

Kinney, J. (2003). *Loosening the grip: A handbook on alcohol information* (7th ed.). New York: McGraw-Hill.

Klatsky, A. L. (1999). Moderate drinking reduced risk of heart disease. *Alcohol Research & Health, 23*(1), 15–24. Retrieved from http://pubs.niaaa.nih.gov/ publications/arh23–1/15–24.pdf

Knapp, C. (1996). *Drinking: A love story.* New York: Dial Press.

Knight, J. R., Wechsler, H., Kuo, M., Seibring, M., Weitzman, E. R., & Schuckit M. (2002). Alcohol abuse and dependence among U.S. college students. *Journal of Studies on Alcohol and Drugs, 63*(3), 263–270.

Kohn, L., Corrigan, J., & Donaldson, M. (Eds.). (2000). *To err is human: Building a safer health system.* Washington, DC: National Academies Press.

Korper, S., & Council, C. (Eds.). (2002). *Substance use by older adults: Estimates of future impact on the treatment system* (DHHS Publication No. SMA 03– 3763, Analytic Series A-21). Rockville, MD: Substance Abuse and Mental Health Services Administration.

Kuo, M., Wechsler, H., Greenberg, P., & Lee, H. (2003). The marketing of alcohol to college students: The role of low prices and special promotions. *American Journal of Preventive Medicine, 25*(3), 204–211.

Kuramoto, F. H. (1995). Asian Americans. In J. Philleo & F. L. Brisbane (Eds.), *Cultural competence for social workers: A guide for alcohol and other drug abuse prevention professionals working with ethnic-racial communities* (DHHS publication No. SMA 95–3075, CSAP Cultural Competence Series No. 4, pp. 105–155). Rockville, MD: U.S. Department of Health and Human Services.

Kurtz, E. (1998). *AA: The story.* San Franciso: Harper and Row.

Kyriacou, D. N., Anglin, D., Taliaferro, E., Stone, S., Tubb, T., Linden, J. A., Muelleman, R., . . . Kraus, J. F. (1999). Risk factors for injury to women from domestic violence. *The New England Journal of Medicine, 341,* 1892–1898.

La Framboise, T. D., Trimble, J. E., & Mohatt, G. V. (1995). Counseling intervention and American Indian tradition: An integrative approach. In R. Hornby (Ed.), *Alcohol and Native Americans* (pp. 149–169). Mission, SD: Sinte Gleska University Press.

Larimer, M. E, Palmer, R. S., & Marlatt, A. (1999). Relapse prevention: An overview of Marlatt's cognitive-behavioral model. *Alcohol Research & Health,
23*(2), 151–159.

Lender, M. E., & Martin, J. K. (1982). *Drinking in America: A history* (Rev. ed.).
New York: Free Press.

Lennard, K. (2008). The role of drinking patterns and acute intoxication in violent
interpersonal behaviors. In International Center for Alcohol Policies (Ed.),
Alcohol and violence: Exploring patterns and responses. Retrieved from
http://ec.europa.eu/health/ph_determinants/life_style/alcohol/Forum/docs/
alcohol_lib18_en.pdf

Lennernäs, H. (2009). Ethanol–drug absorption interaction: Potential for a significant effect on the plasma pharmacokinetics of ethanol vulnerable formu-
lations. *Molecular Pharmaceutics, 6*(5), 1429–1440. Retrieved from http://
pubs.acs.org/doi/full/10.1021/mp9000876

Levine, S. (1984). *Radical departures: Desperate detours to growing up.* New
York: Harcourt.

Liddle, H., & Rowe, C. L. (2006). *Adolescent subtance abuse.* Boston: Cambridge
University Press.

Lieber, C. S. (1999). Microsomal ethanol-oxidizing system (MEOS): The first
30 years (1968–1998)—a review. *Alcoholism: Clinical and Experimental
Research, 23*(6), 991–1007.

Lieber, C. S. (2004). The discovery of the microsomal ethanol oxidizing system
and its physiologic and pathologic role. *Drug Metabolism Reviews, 36*(3–4),
511–529.

Longest, B. (1996). *Seeking strategic advantage through health policy analysis.*
Chicago: Health Administration Press.

Lupton, C., Burd, L., & Harwood, R. (2004). Cost of fetal alcohol spectrum disorders. *American Journal of Medical Genetics, 127C*(1), 42–50.

MacAndrew, C., & Edgerton, R. B. (1969). *Drunken comportment: A social
explanation.* Chicago: Aldine.

MacIntyre, B. (2006, October 21). Bothered and bewildered. *The London Times.*

MacLean, C. (1993). *Scottish toasts and graces.* Belfast: Appletree Press.

Madsen, W. (1967). The alcoholic *agringado. American Anthropologist, 66,* 355–361.

Makela, K. (1986). Attitudes towards drinking and drunkenness in four
Scandanavian cultures. In R. Babor (Ed.), *Annals of the New York Academy
of Sciences: Vol. 472. Alcohol and culture perspectives from Europe and
America* (pp. 21–32). New York: New York Academy of Sciences.

Mann, M. (1958). *Marty Mann's new primer on alcoholism.* New York: Holt,
Rinehart and Winston.

Marczinski, C. A., Harrison, E.L.R., & Fillmore, M. T. (2008). Effects of alcohol
on simulated driving and perceived driving impairment in binge drinkers.
Alcoholism: Clinical and Experimental Research, 32(7), 1329–1337.

Marin Institute. (2009). Alcohol-related harm in the United States. Retrieved from
http://www.marininstitute.org/site/images/stories/pdfs/ftb/Alcohol_Harm.pdf

Marin Institute. (2011). *Alcohol policy.* Retrieved from http://www.marininstitute. org/alcohol_policy

Marlatt, A., & Donovan, D. (2008). *Relapse prevention: Maintenance strategies in the treatment of addictive behaviors.* New York: Guilford Press.

Marsano, L. S., Mendez, C., Hill, D., Barve, S., & McClain, C. J. (2003). Diagnosis and treatment of alcoholic liver disease and its complications. *Alcohol Research & Health, 27*(3), 247–256.

Marshal, M. P., Molina, B.S.G., Pelham, W. E., Jr., & Cheong, J. (2007). Attention-deficit hyperactivity disorder moderates the life stress pathway to alcohol problems in children of alcoholics. *Alcoholism: Clinical and Experimental Research, 31*(4), 564–574.

Marshall, M. (1983). "Four hundred rabbits": An anthropological view of ethanol as a disinhibitor. In R. Room & G. Collins (Eds.), *Alcohol and disinhibition: Nature and meaning of the link* (Research Monograph No. 12; pp. 186–204). Rockville,MD: U.S. Department of Health and Human Services.

Marshall, M. (1991). "Problem deflation" and the ethnographic record: Interpretation and introspection in anthropological studies of alcohol. *Journal of Substance Abuse, 2,* 353–367.

Marshall, M. (Ed.). (1979). *Beliefs, behaviors, and alcoholic beverages: A cross-cultural survey.* Ann Arbor: University of Michigan Press.

Martin, C. S., & Moss, H. B. (1993). Measurement of acute tolerance to alcohol in human subjects. *Alcohol Clinical and Experimental Research, 17*(2), 211–216.

Martin, W. (1986). *The mind of Fredrick Douglass.* Chapel Hill: University of North Carolina Press.

Mathias, R. (1996). Protective factors can buffer high-risk youth from drug use. *NIDA Notes, 11,* 3.

May, P., & Gossage, J. (2001). The epidemiology of alcohol consumption among American Indians living on four reservations and in nearby border towns. *Drug and Alcohol Dependence, 63,* S100.

May, P. A. (1991). Fetal alcohol effects among North American Indians: Evidence and implications for society. *Alcohol Research & Health, 15*(3), 239–248.

May, P. A., Brooke, L., Gossage, J. P., Croxford, J., Adams, C., Jones, K. L.,... Viljoen, D. (2000). Epidemiology of fetal alcohol syndrome in a South African community in the Western Cape Province. *American Journal of Public Health, 90*(12), 1905–1912.

May, P. A., & Gossage, J. P. (2001). Estimating the prevalence of fetal alcohol syndrome: A summary. *Alcohol Research & Health, 25*(3), 159–167.

May, P. A., McCloskey, J., & Gossage, J. P. (2000). *Fetal alcohol syndrome among American Indians: Epidemiology, issues, and research.* NIAAA Research Monographs.

McClellan, T. (2002). Have we evaluated addiction treatment correctly? Implications from a chronic care perspective. *Addiction, 97,* 249–252.

McClelland, G. M., & Teplin, L. A. (2001). Alcohol intoxication and violent crime: Implications for public health policy. *American Journal on Addictions, 10,* 70–85.

McCormick, J. (1984, January 6). Barking up the right tree. *Advertising Age,* 10–12.

McGovern, M. (2003). "The cracked pint glass of the servant: The Irish pub, Irish identity, and the tourist eye. In M. Cronin & B. O'Connor (Eds.), *Irish tourism: Image, culture, and identity.* Clevedon, UK: Channel View.

McGovern, P., Zhang, T., Tang, J., Zhang, Z., Hall, G. R., & Moreau, R. (2004). Fermented beverages of pre- and proto-historic China. *Proceedings of the National Academy of Sciences, 1036,* 278–289.

McLean, S. A., Blow, F. C., Walton, M. A., Barry, K. L., Maio, R. F., & Knutzen, S. R. (2003). At risk drinking among injured older adults presenting to the emergency department. *Academy of Emergency Medicine, 10*(5), 536.

Merck. (2011). *The Merck manuals online medical library: Manifestations of liver disease: Portal hypertension.* Whitehouse Station, NJ: Author. Retrieved from http://www.merckmanuals.com/home/sec10/ch135/ch135d.html

Mignon, S. I., Faiia, M. M., Myers, P. L., & Rubington, E. (2009). *Substance use and abuse: Exploring alcohol and drug issues.* Boulder, CO: Lynne Reinner.

Miller, B. A., Downs, W. R., & Testa, M. (1993). Interrelationships between victimization experiences and women's alcohol use. *Journal of Studies on Alcohol and Drugs* (Suppl. 11), 109–117.

Miller, B. A., Maguin, E., & Down, W. R. (1997). Alcohol, drugs, and violence in children's lives. In M. Galanter (Ed.), *Recent developments in alcoholism: Alcoholism and violence* (Vol. 13; pp. 357–385). New York: Plenum Press.

Miller, L. C., Chan, W., Litvinova, A., Rubin, A., Comfort, K., Tirella, L., . . . Kovalev, I. (2006). Fetal alcohol spectrum disorders in children residing in Russian orphanages: A phenotypic survey. *Alcoholism: Clinical and Experimental Research, 30*(3), 531–538.

Miller, W., & Willbourne, P. (n.d.). *Whatever happened to controlled drinking?* Poster session, University of New Mexico Center on Alcoholism, Substance Abuse, and Addictions (CASAA), Albuquerque, NM. Retrieved from http://casaa.unm.edu/posters/Whatever%20Happened%20to%20Controlled%20Drinking.pdf

Miller, W. R., & Rollnick, S. (1991). *Motivational interviewing: Preparing people to change addictive behavior.* New York: Guilford Press.

Minuchin, S. (1974). *Families and family therapy.* Cambridge, MA: Harvard University Press.

Minuchin, S., & Fishman, H. C. (1981). *Family therapy techniques.* Cambridge, MA: Harvard University Press.

Misch, D. (2007). Natural recovery from alcohol abuse among college students. *Journal of American College Health, 55*(4), 215–218.

Molina, B.S.G., & Pelham, W. E., Jr. (2003). Childhood predictors of adolescent substance use in a longitudinal study of children with ADHD. *Journal of Abnormal Psychology, 112*(3), 497–507.

Moos, R., Brennan, P., & Schutte, K. (1998). Life context factors, treatment, and late-life drinking behavior. In E.S.L. Gomberg, A. M. Hegedus, & R. A. Zucker (Eds.), *Alcohol problems and aging* (NIAAA Research Monograph No. 33. NIH Pub. No. 98-4163). Bethesda, MD: NIAAA.

Moos, R., Brennan, P., Schutte, K., & Moos, B. (2004). High-risk alcohol consumption and late-life alcohol use problems. *American Journal of Public Health, 94,* 1985–1991.

Moos, R., & Holahan, C. (2010). Social and financial resources and high-risk alcohol consumption among older adults. *Alcoholism Clinical and Experimental Research, 34*(4), 646–654.

Moskowitz, H., Burns, M. M., & Williams, A. F. (1985). Skills performance at low blood alcohol levels. *Journal of Studies on Alcohol and Drugs, 46,* 482–485.

Mothers Against Drunk Driving. (2011). The Support 21 Coalition. Retrieved from http://www.why21.org

Muehlfried, F. (2006). Food chains sharing the same blood: Culture and cuisine in the Republic of Georgia. *Food Anthropology,* S3.

Murray, C. J., & Lopez, A. D. (1996). *The global burden of disease.* Boston, MA: Harvard School of Public Health.

Myers, P. L. (1983, September). Cautionary notes on ethnic/psychiatric stereotypes. *Medical Tribune.*

Myers, P. L. (1990). Sources and configurations of institutional denial. *Employee Assistance Quarterly, 5*(3), 43–54.

Myers, P. L. (2002). The management of identity in bodegas: Stigma and microeconomics in Brooklyn. *Journal of Ethnicity in Substance Abuse, 1*(3), 75–92.

Myers, P. L. (2008). Borderline personality disorder as a co-occurring disorder. In G. Fischer & N. Roget (Eds.), *Encyclopedia of substance abuse prevention, treatment, and recovery.* Thousand Oaks, CA: Sage Publications.

Myers, P. L., & Salt, N. R. (2007). *Becoming an addictions counselor: A comprehensive text* (2nd ed.). Sudbury, MA: Jones and Bartlett.

National Council on Alcoholism and Drug Dependence. (1990). *Definition of alcoholism.* Retrieved from http://www.ncadd.org/facts/defalc.html

National Highway Traffic Safety Administration. (1989). *The impact of minimum drinking age laws on fatal crash involvements: An update of the NHTSA analyses* (NHTSA Technical Report, No. DOT HS 807 349). Washington, DC: National Highway Traffic Safety Administration.

National Highway Traffic Safety Administration. (1994). *A preliminary assessment of the lowering of the BAC per se limit in five states.* Washington, DC: National Highway Safety Transportation Administration. Retrieved from http://www-nrd.nhtsa.dot.gov/Pubs/BAC08RPT.PDF

National Highway Traffic Safety Administration. (2000a). *A review of the literature on the effects of low doses of alcohol on driving related skills.* Washington, DC: National Highway Traffic Safety Administration.

National Highway Traffic Safety Administration. (2000b). *On DWI laws in other countries.* Retrieved from http://www.nhtsa.dot.gov/people/injury/research/pub/dwiothercountries/dwiothercountries.html

National Highway Traffic Safety Administration. (2009b). *2008 traffic safety annual assessment: Highlights.* Retrieved from http://www-nrd.nhtsa.dot.gov/Pubs/811172.pdf

National Institute on Alcohol Abuse and Alcoholism. (1994). *Alcohol and hormones* (Alcohol Alert No. 26). Retrieved from http://pubs.niaaa.nih.gov/publications/aa26.htm

National Institute on Alcohol Abuse and Alcoholism. (1995a). *Alcohol-medication interactions* (Alcohol Alert No. 27). Retrieved from http://pubs.niaaa.nih.gov/publications/aa27.htm

National Institute on Alcohol Abuse and Alcoholism. (1995b). *College drinking* (Alcohol Alert No. 29 PH 357).

National Institute of Alcohol Abuse and Alcoholism. (1998a). *Alcohol and aging* (Alcohol Alert No. 40). Retrieved from http://pubs.niaaa.nih.gov/publications/aa40.htm

National Institute on Alcohol Abuse and Alcoholism. (1999a). *Alcohol and the workplace* (Alcohol Alert No. 44).

National Institute on Alcohol Abuse and Alcoholism. (1999b). (Alcohol Alert No. 46).

National Institute on Alcohol Abuse and Alcoholism (2000). *Issues in fetal alcohol syndrome prevention. Tenth special report to the U.S. Congress on alcohol and health.*

National Institute on Alcohol Abuse and Alcoholism. (2002). *Alcohol and AIDS* (Alcohol Alert No. 57). Retrieved from http://pubs.niaaa.nih.gov/publications/aa57.htm

National Institute on Alcohol Abuse and Alcoholism. (2004a). *Alcohol: An important women's health issue* (Alcohol Alert No. 62). Rockville, MD: U.S. HHS, PHS, NIAAA.

National Institute on Alcohol Abuse and Alcoholism. (2004b). NIAAA council approves definition of binge drinking. *NIAAA Newsletter* (winter), 3.

National Institute on Alcohol Abuse and Alcoholism. (2010a). *Alcohol policy information system: Alcohol policy at a glance.* Retrieved from http://alcoholpolicy.niaaa.nih.gov/APIS_policy_changes.html

National Institute on Alcohol Abuse and Alcoholism. (2010b). *College drinking: Changing the culture.* Retrieved from http://www.collegedrinkingprevention.gov/NIAAACollegeMaterials/TaskForce/Issues_00.aspx

National Survey on Drug Use and Health. (2004, August 20). *Women with co-occurring serious mental illness and a substance use disorder.* Retrieved from http://www.oas.samhsa.gov/2k4/femDual/femDual.htm

National Survey on Drug Use and Health. (2005, April 1). *Alcohol and delinquent behavior among youth.* Retrieved from http://oas.samhsa.gov/2k5/alcDelinquent/alcDelinquent.pdf

National Survey on Drug Use and Health. (2007). *Gender differences in alcohol use and alcohol dependence or abuse: 2004 and 2005.* Retrieved from http://www.oas.samhsa.gov/2k7/AlcGender/AlcGender.htm

NBC News. (2008). Tragedy at Pine Ridge. Retrieved from http://icue.nbcunifiles.com/icue/files/icue/site/pdf/36485.pdf

Netting, R. (1964). Beer as a locus of value among the West African Kofyar. *American Anthropologist, 66*(2), 375–384.

New York Times. (1922, September 12). Denatured alcohol blamed for deaths. *The New York Times.* Retrieved from http://query.nytimes.com/mem/archive-free/pdf?_r=1&res=9501EEDF1F3AE433A25753C1A96F9C946395D6CF

New York Times. (1990, December 11). Doctors criticized on fetal problem. *The New York Times.* Retrieved from http://www.nytimes.com/1990/12/11/us/doctors-criticized-on-fetal-problem.html?pagewanted=1

Newlin, D. B., & Thomson, J. B. (1990). Alcohol challenge with sons of alcoholics: A critical review and analysis. *Psychological Bulletin, 108*(3), 383–402.

Newport, M. (2010, August 7). U.S. drinking rate edges up slightly to 25-year high. Retrieved from http://www.gallup.com/poll/141656/Drinking-Rate-Edges-Slightly-Year-High.aspx?utm_source=email%2Ba%2Bfriend&utm_medium=email&utm_campaign=sharing&utm_term=Drinking-Rate-Edges-Slightly-Year-High&utm_content=morelink

Nielsen, A. (2000). Examining drinking patterns and problems among Hispanic groups: Results from a national survey. *Journal of Studies on Alcohol, 2,* 301–10.

North-American Interfraternity Council. (2009). *Resolutions of the House of Delegates: Alcohol.* Retrieved from http://www.nicindy.org/about/resolutions/#Alcohol%20Education

Nurnberger, J. I., Jr., & Bierut, L. J. (2007). The genetics of alcoholism. *Scientific American, 296*(4), 46–53.

Nuwer, G. (1999). *Wrongs of passage: Fraternities, sororities, hazing, and binge drinking.* Bloomington: Indiana University Press.

O'Carroll, C. (2006). Cold beer, warm hearts: Community, belonging, and desire in Irish pubs in Berlin. In T. W. Wilson (Ed.), *Drinking cultures.* Oxford: Berg.

Oldenburg, R. (1999). *The great good place.* New York: Marlowe & Company.

O'Malley, P. M., & Johnston, L. D. (2002). Epidemiology of alcohol and other drug use among American college students. *Journal of Studies on Alcohol and Drugs* (Suppl. 14), 23–39.

O'Malley, P. M., & Wagenaar, A. C. (1991). Effects of minimum drinking age laws on alcohol use, related behaviors, and traffic crash involvement among American youth: 1976–1987. *Journal of Studies on Alcohol and Drugs, 52,* 478–491.

Oscar-Berman, M., & Marinkovic, K. (2003). Alcoholism and the brain: An overview. *Alcohol Research & Health, 27*(2), 125–133. Retrieved from http://pubs.niaaa.nih.gov/publications/arh27–2/125–133.pdf

Oxford House. (2011). Oxford House Movement. Retrieved from http://www.oxfordhouse.org/

Pacific Institute for Research and Evaluation. (2009). *Underage drinking costs.* Retrieved from http://www.udetc.org/UnderageDrinkingCosts.asp

Pagano, M. E., Rende, R., Rodriguez, B. F., Hargraves, E. L., Moskowitz, A. T., & Keller, M. B. (2007). Impact of parental history of substance use disorders on the clinical course of anxiety disorders. *Substance Abuse Treatment, Prevention, and Policy, 2,* 13.

Park, A., Sher, K. J., Wood, P. K., & Krull, J. L. (2009). Dual mechanisms underlying accentuation of risky drinking via fraternity/sorority affiliation: The role of personality, peer norms, and alcohol availability. *Journal of Abnormal Psychology, 118*(2), 241–255.

Park, S-Y., Shibusawa, T., Yoon, S. M., & Son, H. (2010). Characteristics of Chinese and Korean Americans in outpatient treatment for alcohol use disorders: Examining heterogeneity among Asian American subgroups. *Journal of Ethnicity in Substance Abuse, 9, 2.*

Parker, L. L., Penton-Voak, I. S., Attwood, A. A., & Munafo, M. R. (2008). Effects of acute alcohol consumption on ratings of attractiveness of facial stimuli: Evidence of long-term encoding. *Alcohol and Alcoholism, 43*(6), 636–640.

Peele, S. (1992, March). Review of the book *Alcohol and the addictive brain. Reason,* 51–54. Retrieved from http://www.peele.net/lib/blumrev.html

Pegram, T. R. (1998). *Battling demon rum: The struggle for a dry America.* Chicago: Ivan R. Dee.

Perkins, H. W. (Ed.). (2003). *The social norms approach to preventing school and college age substance abuse.* San Francisco: Jossey-Bass.

Perkins, H. W., & Craig, D. W. (2003). The imaginary lives of peers: Patterns of substance use and misperceptions of norms among secondary school students. In H. W. Perkins (Ed.), *The social norms approach to preventing school and college substance abuse: A handbook for educators, counselors, and clinicians.* San Francisco: Jossey-Bass.

Perrine, M. W. (1990). Who are the drinking drivers? The spectrum of drinking drivers revisited. *Alcohol Health and Research World, 14,* 26–35.

Pettinati, H. M., Oslin, D. W., Kampman, K. M., Dundon, W. D., Xie, H., Gallis, T. L., Dackis, C. A., & O'Brien, C. P. (2010). A double-blind, placebo-controlled trial combining Sertraline and Naltrexone for treating co-occurring depression and alcohol dependence. *American Journal of Psychiatry, 167,* 668–675.

Pletcher, M. J., Maselli, J., & Gonzales, R. (2004). Uncomplicated alcohol intoxication in the emergency department: An analysis of the National Hospital Ambulatory Medical Care Survey. *American Journal of Medicine, 117,* 863.

Presley, C. A., Leichliter, J. S., & Meilman, P. W. (1995). *Alcohol and drugs on American college campuses: A report to college presidents: Third in a series, 1995, 1996, and 1997.* Carbondale: Southern Illinois University.

Preuss, U. W., Koller, G., Barnow, S., Eikmeier, M., & Soyka, M. (2006). Suicidal behavior in alcohol-dependent subjects: The role of personality disorders. *Alcohol: Clinical and Experimental Research, 30*(5), 866–877.

Primack, B. A., Dalton, M. A., Carroll, M. V., Agarwal, A. A., & Fine, M. J. (2008). Content analysis of tobacco, alcohol, and other drugs in popular music. *Archives of Pediatriatrics & Adolescent Medicine, 162*(2), 169–175.

Prochaska, J. O., & DiClemente, C. C. (1982). Transtheoretical therapy: Toward a more integrative model of change. *Psychotherapy: Theory, Research and Practice, 19*(3), 276–288.

Prochaska, J. O., Norcross, J., & DiClemente, C. C. (1994). *Changing for good.* New York: Avon Books.

Randall, C. L., Roberts, J. S., Del Boca, F. K., Carroll, K. M., Connors, G. J., & Mattson, M. E. (1999). Telescoping of landmark events associated with drinking: A gender comparison. *Journal of Studies on Alcohol, 60*(2), 252–260.

Rehm, J. (2009). Commentary: Alcohol poisoning in Russia: Implications for monitoring and comparative risk factor assessment. *International Journal of Epidemiology, 38*(1), 154–155.

Rehm, J., Mathers, C., Popova, S., Thavorncharoensap, M., Teerawattananon, Y., & Patra, J. (2009). Global burden of disease and injury and economic cost attributable to alcohol use and alcohol-use disorders. *Lancet, 373*(9682), 2223–2233.

Rehm, J., Rehn, N., Room, R., Monteiro, M., Gmel, G., Jernigan, D., & Frick, U. (2003). The global distribution of average volume of alcohol consumption and patterns of drinking. *European Addiction Research, 9,* 147–156.

Reich, T., Hinrichs, A., Culverhouse, R., & Bierut, L. (1999). Genetic studies of alcoholism and substance dependence. *American Journal of Human Genetics, 65,* 599–605.

Reidy, C. (1990, August 26). Kitty Dukakis fled "depression" in binges, book says. *The Boston Globe.*

Reynolds, K., Lewis, L. B., Nolen, J. D., Kinney, G. L., Sathya, B., & He, J. (2003). Alcohol consumption and risk of stroke: A meta-analysis. *Journal of the American Medical Association, 289,* 579–588.

Ricourt, M., & Danta, R. (2003). *Hispanas de Queens: Latino panethnicity in a New York City neighborhood.* Ithaca, NY: Cornell University Press.

Roberts, C., & Robinson, S. P. (2007). Alcohol concentration and carbonation of drinks: The effect on blood alcohol levels. *Journal of Forensic Legal Medicine, 4*(7), 398–405.

Roche, A. M, & Freeman, T. (2004). Brief interventions: Good in theory but weak in practice. *Drug and Alcohol Review, 23,* 11–18.

Roebuck, T. M., Mattson, S. N., & Riley, E. P. (1999). Behavioral and psychosocial profiles of alcohol-exposed children. *Alcohol: Clinical and Experiment Research, 23,* 1070–1076.

Roehrs, T., & Roth, T. (2001). Sleep, sleepiness, and alcohol use. *Alcohol Research & Health, 25*(2), 101–109.

Rohrabough, W. J. (1979). *The alcoholic republic: An American tradition.* Oxford: Oxford University Press.

Room, R. (1984). Alcohol and ethnography: A case of problem deflation? *Current Anthropology, 25*(2), 169–191.

Rosenquist, J. N., Murabito, J., Fowler, J. H., & Christakis, N. A. (2010). The spread of alcohol consumption behavior in a large social network. *Annals of Internal Medicine, 152*(7), 426–433.

Rotgers, F., Kern, M. F., & Hoeltzel, R. (2002). *Responsible drinking: A moderation management approach for problem drinkers.* Oakland, CA: New Harbinger.

Rubel, A. J. (1984). *Susto: A folk illness.* Berkeley: University of California Press.

Rubin, E., & Doria, J. (1990). Alcoholic cardiomyopathy: Alcohol as a cause of heart muscle disease. *Alcohol Research & Health, 14*(4), 277–284.

Sanchez-Craig, M., Wilkinson, D. A., & Davila, R. (1995). Empirically based guidelines for moderate drinking: 1-year results from three studies with problem drinkers. *American Journal of Public Health, 85*(6), 823–828.

Sargent, M. J. (1967). Changes in Japanese drinking patterns. *Quarterly Journal of Studies on Alcohol, 28,* 709–722.

Satir, V. (1964). *Conjoint family therapy.* Palo Alto, CA: Science and Behavior Books.

Schuckit, M., Rimmer, J., Reich, T., & Winokur, G. (1971). The bender alcoholic. *The British Journal of Psychiatry, 119,* 183–184.

Schuckit, M. A. (2009). An overview of genetic influences in alcoholism. *Journal of Substance Abuse Treatment, 36*(1), s5–s14.

Schwartz, J. (2008). Gender differences in drunk driving prevalence rates and trends: A 20-year assessment using multiple sources of evidence. *Addictive Behaviors, 33*(9), 1217–1222.

Schwartz, J., & Rookey, B. D. (2006). *DUI arrest patterns have changed, but has DUI behavior?: Sex-by-age disaggregated trends in drunk driving in the US, 1980–2000.* Paper presented at the annual meeting of the American Society of Criminology, Los Angeles Convention Center, Los Angeles.

Scribner, R. A., MacKinnon, D. P., & Dwyer, J. H. (1995). The risk of assaultive violence and alcohol availability in Los Angeles County. *American Journal of Public Health, 3*(85), 335–340.

Seligman, M.E.P. (1975). *Helplessness: On depression, development, and death.* San Francisco: Freeman.

Seto, M. C., & Barbaree, H. E. (1997). Sexual aggression as antisocial behavior: A developmental model. In D.M. Stoff, J. Breiling, & J.D. Maser (Eds.), *Handbook of antisocial behavior* (pp. 524–533). New York: Wiley.

Sher, L. (2005). Alcohol consumption and suicide. *Quarterly Journal of Medicine, 99*(1), 57–61.

Siebert, D., Wilke, D., Delva, J., Smith, M. R., & Howell, R. L. (2003). Differences in African American and white college students' drinking behaviors: Consequences, harm reduction strategies, and health information sources. *Journal of American College Health, 52*(3), 123–129.

Simboli, B. J. (1984). Acculturated Italian-American drinking behavior. In L. A. Bennett & G. M. Ames (Eds.), *The American experience with alcohol* (pp. 61–76). New York: Plenum Press.

Skodol, A. E., Gunderson, J. G., Pfohl, B., Widiger, T. A., Livesley, W. J., & Siever, L. J. (2002). The borderline diagnosis II: Biology, genetics, and clinical course. *Biological Psychiatry, 51*(12), 951–963.

Smith, B. H., Molina, B.S.G., & Pelham, W. E., Jr. (2002). The clinically meaningful link between alcohol use and attention deficit hyperactivity disorder. *Alcohol Research and Health, 26*(2), 122–129. Retrieved from http://pubs.niaaa.nih.gov/publications/arh26–2/122–129.pdf

Smith, C., Lizotte, A. J., Thornberry, T. P., & Krohn M. D. (1995). Resilient youth: Identifying factors that prevent high-risk youth from engaging in delinquency and drug use. In J. Hagan (Ed.), *Delinquency and disrepute in the life course* (pp. 217–247). Greenwich, CT: JAI Press.

Smith, M. J., Barch, D. M., Wolf, T. J., Mamah, D., & Csernansky, J. G. (2008). Elevated rates of substance use disorders in non-psychotic siblings of individuals with schizophrenia. *Schizophrenia Research, 106*(2/3), 294–299.

Smith, W. (2010). *Alcohol abuse and the elderly: The hidden population.* Retrieved from http://ezinearticles.com/?Alcohol-Abuse-and-the-Elderly:-The-Hidden-Population&id=227801.

Sonne, S. C., & Brady, K. T. (2001). *Bipolar disorder and alcoholism.* Retrieved from http://pubs.niaaa.nih.gov/publications/arh26–2/103–108.htm

Spindler, G., & Spindler, L. (1971). *Dreamers without power: The Menomini Indians.* New York: Holt, Rinehart, and Winston.

Starner, T. (2010, February 10). *Scared of the stigma.* Human Resources Executive Online. Retrieved from http://www.hreonline.com/HRE/story.jsp?story Id=338924508

Steinberg, N. (1999). *Drunkard: A hard drinking life.* New York: Plume/Penguin Group.

Stickley, A., Leinsalu, M., Andreev, E., Razvodovsky, Y., Vågerö, D., & McKee, M. (2007). Alcohol poisoning in Russia and the countries in the European part of the former Soviet Union, 1970–2002. *The European Journal of Public Health, 17*(5), 444–449.

Stolberg, V. (1993). Alcohol and drug usage by New Jersey college students. *National Social Science Perspectives Journal, 3*(1), 266–275.

Stolberg, V. (2010). International Coalition for Addiction studies member listserv.

Stoner, S. A., George, W. H., Norris, J., & Peters, L. M. (2007). Liquid courage: Alcohol fosters risky sexual decision-making in individuals with sexual fears. *AIDS and Behavior, 11,* 217–226.

Stout, R. L., Rubin, A., Zwick, W., Zywiak, W., & Bellino, L. (1999). Optimizing the cost-effectiveness of alcohol treatment: A rationale for extended case monitoring. *Addictive Behaviors, 24*(1, 2), 17–35.

Stratton K., Howe, C., & Battaglia, F., eds. (1996). *Fetal alcohol syndrome: Diagnosis, epidemiology, prevention and treatment.* Washington, DC: National Academic Press.

Streissguth, A. (1994). A long-term perspective of FAS. *Alcohol Research & Health, 18*(1), 74–81.

Streissguth, A. P., Barr, H. M., & Kogan, J., & Bookstein, F. L. (1996). *Understanding the occurrence of secondary disabilities in clients with fetal alcohol syndrome (FAS) and fetal alcohol effects (FAE): Final report to the Centers for Disease Control and Prevention (CDC)* (Tech. Rep. No. 96–06). Seattle: University of Washington Fetal Alcohol & Drug Unit.

Strom, S. (2010, June 18). Nonprofit advocate carves out a for-profit niche. *The New York Times,* p. A10. Retrieved from http://www.nytimes.com/2010/06/18/us/politics/18berman.html

Su, S. S., Larison, C., Ghadialy, R., Johnson, R., & Rohde, F. (1997, September). *Substance use among women in the United States* (DHHS Publication No. SMA 97-3162). Rockville, MD: Office of Applied Studies, Substance Abuse and Mental Health Services Administration.

Substance Abuse and Mental Health Services Administration. (1997). *Risk and protective factors for adolescent substance abuse: Findings from the 1997 National Household Survey on Drug Abuse.* Retrieved from http://www.oas.samhsa.gov/NHSDA/NAC97/Table_of_Contents.htm

Substance Abuse and Mental Health Services Administration. (1998). *OAS data systems and publications.* Retrieved from http://www.oas.samhsa.gov/systems.htm

Substance Abuse and Mental Health Services Administration (2006a). *Addiction counseling competencies: The knowledge, skills, and attitudes of professional practice* (DHHS Publication No. SMA 06-4171). Rockville, MD: Substance Abuse and Mental Health Services Administration.

Substance Abuse and Mental Health Services Administration. (2006b). *Results from the 2005 National Survey on Drug Use and Health: National findings* (Office of Applied Studies, NSDUH Series H-30, DHHS Publication No. SMA 06-4194). Rockville, MD. Retrieved from http://www.oas.samhsa.gov/nsduh/2k5nsduh/2k5results.htm

Substance Abuse and Mental Health Services Administration. (2007). *Sexually transmitted diseases and substance abuse.* Retrieved from http://oas.samhsa.gov/2k7/STD/STD.htm

Substance Abuse Mental Health Services Administration. (2009). *Substance abuse prevention dollars and cents: A cost-benefit analysis.* Retrieved from http://download.ncadi.samhsa.gov/prevline/pdfs/SMA07–4298.pdf

Substance Abuse and Mental Health Services Administration. (n.d.). *PTSD and alcohol fact sheet.* Retrieved from http://www.samhsa.gov/csatdisaster recovery/outreach/ptsdAndProblemsWithAlcohol.pdf

Taleff, M. J. (1994). The well-deserved death of denial. *Behavioral Health Management, 14*(3), 51–52.

Thom, B. (2003). *Risk-taking behaviour in men: Substance use and gender.* London: Health Development Agency.

Thomas, S. E., Kelly, S. J., Mattson, S. N., & Riley, E. P. (1998). Comarison of social abilities of children with fetal alcohol syndrome to those of children with similar IQ scores and normal controls. *Alcohol: Clinical and Experimental Research, 22,* 528–533.

Thorogood, G. (2007) "One Bourbon, One Scotch, One Beer," performed by George Thorogood & The Destroyers (Rounder CD-3013).

Toombs, R. (1953). "One Bourbon, One Scotch, One Beer," performed by Champion Jack Dupree in 1975. Retrieved from http://www.youtube.com/watch?v=o5SozTlkqas

Transportation Research Board. (2003). *Implementing impaired driving countermeasures* (Transportation Research Circular E-C072). Washington, DC: Author.

Tsai, V. W., Anderson, C. L., & Vaca, F. E. (2010). Alcohol involvement among young female drivers in US fatal crashes: Unfavourable trends. *Injury Prevention, 16,* 17–20.

University of Washington. (2011). *Liver and ascites.* Seattle: University of Washington Department of Medicine. Accessed January 9, 2011, from http://depts.washington.edu/physdx/liver/index.html

Unwin, T. (1991). *Wine and the vine: An historical geography of viticulture and the wine trade.* London: Routledge.

U.S. Surgeon General. (2007). *Call to action to prevent and reduce underage drinking.* Retrieved from http://www.surgeongeneral.gov/topics/underage drinking/calltoaction.pdf

Van Gennep, A. (1960). *The rites of passage.* Chicago: University of Chicago Press.

Velasquez, M. M., Maurer, G. G., Crouch, C., & DiClemente, C. C. (2001). *Group treatment for substance abuse: A stages-of-change therapy manual.* New York: The Guilford Press.

Vinson, D. C., Galliher, J. M., Reidinger, C., & Kappus, J. A. (2004). Comfortably engaging: Which approach to alcohol screening should we use? *Annals of Family Medicine, 2*(5), 398–404.

Wagenaar, A. C. (1983). *Alcohol, young drivers, and traffic accidents.* Lexington, MA: Lexington Books.

Wagenaar, A. C. (1993). Minimum drinking age and alcohol availability to youth: Issues and research needs. In M. E. Hilton & G. Bloss G (Eds.), *Economics and the prevention of alcohol-related problems* (Research Monograph No. 25, NIH Pub. No. 93–3513, pp. 175–200). Bethesda, MD: National Institute on Alcohol Abuse and Alcoholism.

Wallace, A.F.C. (1956). Revitalization movements. *American Anthropologist, 58,* 264–281.

Wallace, A.F.C., & Steen, S. C. (1970). *The death and rebirth of the Seneca.* New York: Random House.

Weathermon, R., & Crabb, D. W. (1999). Alcohol and medication interactions. *Alcohol Research & Health, 23*(1), 40–54.

Wechsler, H., Davenport, A., Dowdall, G., Moeykens, B., & Castillo, S. (1994). Health and behavioral consequences of binge drinking in college: A national survey of students at 140 campuses. *Journal of the American Medical Society, 272,* 1672–1677.

Wechsler, H., & Isaac, N. (1992). "Binge" drinkers at colleges: Prevalence, drinking time, time trends, and associated problems. *Journal of the American Medical Association, 267,* 2929–2931.

Wechsler, H., Kuh, G. D., & Davenport, A. (1996). Fraternities, sororities, and binge drinking: Results from a national study of American colleges. *NASPA Journal, 33*(4), 260–279.

Wechsler, H., & Kuo, M. (2000). College students define binge drinking and estimate its prevalence: Results of a national survey. *Journal of American College Health, 49*(2), 57–64.

Wechsler, H., & Kuo, M. (2003). Watering down the drinks: The moderating effect of college demographics on alcohol use of high-risk groups. *American Journal of Public Health, 93*(11), 1929–1933.

Wechsler, H., Nelson, T. F., Lee, J. E., Seibring, M., Lewis, C., & Keeling, R. P (2003). Perception and reality: A national evaluation of social norms marketing interventions to reduce college students' heavy alcohol use. *Journal of Studies on Alcohol and Drugs, 63*(4), 484–494.

Wechsler, H., & Nelson, T. F. (2008). What we have learned from the Harvard School of Public Health College Alcohol Study: Focusing attention on college student alcohol consumption and the environmental conditions that promote it. *Journal of Studies on Alcohol and Drugs, 69*(4), 481–490.

Wechsler, H., & Sands, E.S. (1980). Minimum-age laws and youthful drinking: An introduction. In H. Wechsler (Ed.), *Minimum drinking age laws* (pp. 1–10). Lexington, MA: Lexington Books.

Wechsler, H., & Wuethrich, B. (2002). *Dying to drink: Confronting binge drinking on college campuses.* Rodale Press.

Weinberg, N. (2001). Risk factors for adolescent substance abuse. *Journal of Learning Disabilities, 34*(4), 343–351.

Wells, R., Lemak, C., Alexander, J., Nahra, T., Ye, Y., & Campbell, C. (2007). Do licensing and accreditation matter in outpatient substance abuse treatment programs? *Journal of Substance Abuse Treatment, 33*(1), 43–50.

West, M., & Prinz, R. (1987). Parental alcoholism and childhood psychopathology. *Psychological Bulletin, 102,* 204–218.

White, A. M. (2003). What happened?: Alcohol, memory blackouts, and the brain. *Alcohol Research & Health, 27*(2), 186–196.

White, A. M., Jamieson-Drake, D. W., & Swartzwelder, H. S. (2002). Prevalence and correlates of alcohol-induced blackouts among college students: Results of an e–mail survey. *Journal of American College Health, 51,* 117–131.

White, W. I. (1998). *Slaying the dragon: The history of sddiction treatment and recovery in America.* Bloomington, IN: Chestnut Health Systems.

White Bison. (2002). *The red road to wellbriety—in the Native American way.* Colorado Springs, CO: White Bison.

Whitehead, P. C. (1977). *Alcohol and young drivers: Impact and implications of lowering the drinking age.* Ottawa: Department of National Health and Welfare.

Whitehead, P. C., Craig, J., Langford, N., MacArthur, C., Stanton, B., & Ferrence, R. G. (1975). Collision behavior of young drivers: Impact of the change in the age of majority. *Journal of Studies on Alcohol and Drugs, 36,* 1208–1223.

Widom, C. S., & Hiller-Sturmhofel, S. (2001). Alcohol abuse as a risk factor for and consequence of child abuse. *Alcohol Research & Health, 25*(1), 52–57.

Widom, C. S., White, H. R., Czaja, S. L., & Marmorstein, N. R. (2007). Long-term effects of child abuse and neglect on alcohol use and excessive drinking in middle adulthood. *Journal of Studies on Alcohol and Drugs, 68*(3), 317–316.

Wilder-Taylor, S. (2006). *Sippy cups are not for chardonnay.* New York: Simon Spotlight Entertainment.

Wilder-Taylor, S. (2008). *Nap time is the new happy hour.* New York: Simon Spotlight Entertainment.

Williams, A. F., Rich, R. F., Zador, P. L., & Robertson, L. S. (1974). The legal minimum drinking age and fatal motor vehicle crashes. Washington, DC: Insurance Institute for Highway Safety.

Williamson, R. J., Sham, P., & Ball, P. (2003). Binge drinking trends in a UK community-based sample. *Journal of Substance Use, 8*(4), 234–237.

Wilsnack, S. C., Vogeltanz, N. D., Klassen, A. D., & Harris, T. R. (1997). Childhood sexual abuse and women's substance abuse: National survey findings. *Journal of Studies on Alcohol and Drugs, 58*(3), 264–271.

Windle, M., & Searles, J. S. (1990). *Children of alcoholics: Critical perspectives.* New York: Guilford Press.

Winick, J. C. (1962). Maturing out of narcotics addiction. *Bulletin on Narcotics, 6,* 1.

World Health Organization. (2004). *World Health Organization global status report on alcohol 2004.* Geneva: Author.

World Health Organization. (2010a). *Alcohol.* Retrieved from http://www.who.int/substance_abuse/facts/alcohol/en/index.html

World Health Organization. (2010b). *Working document for developing a draft global strategy to reduce harmful use of alcohol.* Retrieved from http://www.who.int/substance_abuse/activities/msbwden.pdf

Wutzke, S. E., Conigrave, K. M., Saunders, J.A.B., & Hall, W. D. (2002). The long-term effectiveness of brief interventions for unsafe alcohol consumption: A 10-year follow-up. *Addiction, 97,* 665–675.

Wylie, L. (1964). *Village in the Vaucluse.* New York: Harper Colophon Books.

Yalisove, D. (2004). *Alcohol research.* Boston: Pearson Education.

Yalisove, D. L. (1998). The origins and evolution of the disease concept of treatment. *Journal of Studies on Alcohol and Drugs, 59,* 469–476.

Zador, P. L. (1991). Alcohol–related relative risk of fatal driver injuries in relation to driver age and sex. *Journal of Studies on Alcohol, 52*(4), 302–310.

Zaridze, D., Maximovitch, D., Lazarev, A., Igitov, V., Boroda, A., Boreham, J. . . . Boffetta, P. (2009). Alcohol poisoning is a main determinant of recent mortality trends in Russia: Evidence from a detailed analysis of mortality statistics and autopsies. *International Journal of Epidemiology, 38*(1), 143–153.

Zealberg, J., & Brady, K. (1999). Substance abuse and emergency psychiatry. *Psychiatric Clinics of North America, 22*(4), 803–817.

INDEX

About the Authors

Peter L. Myers, professor emeritus of addiction studies, is editor of the *Journal of Ethnicity in Substance Abuse* and past president of the International Coalition for Addiction Studies Education. Myers is author of numerous books and publications on drug abuse and abuse. He is a member of the new National Addiction Studies Accreditation Commission, LLC.

Richard E. Isralowitz, PhD, is professor and director of the Regional Alcohol and Drug Abuse Resources Center at Ben Gurion University. Isralowitz is author of numerous books and publications on drug use and abuse; he is a Fulbright Scholar and a Distinguished International Scientist with the National Institute on Drug Abuse.